Crystal and Stone Massage

"*Crystal and Stone Massage* is the standard work in the field of gentle massage with precious stones. The authors are outstanding in their ability to convey the energetic aspects of massage and the importance of touch. Six different massage techniques are illustrated in detail, from intuitive massages to very complex reflexology. . . . Recommended for both professional massage therapists as well as the layperson."

DAGMAR FLECK,
COAUTHOR OF *HOT STONE AND GEM MASSAGE*

"An excellent overview and introduction to the various methods and techniques of massage using crystals."

FRED HAGENEDER,
AUTHOR OF *THE MEANING OF TREES*

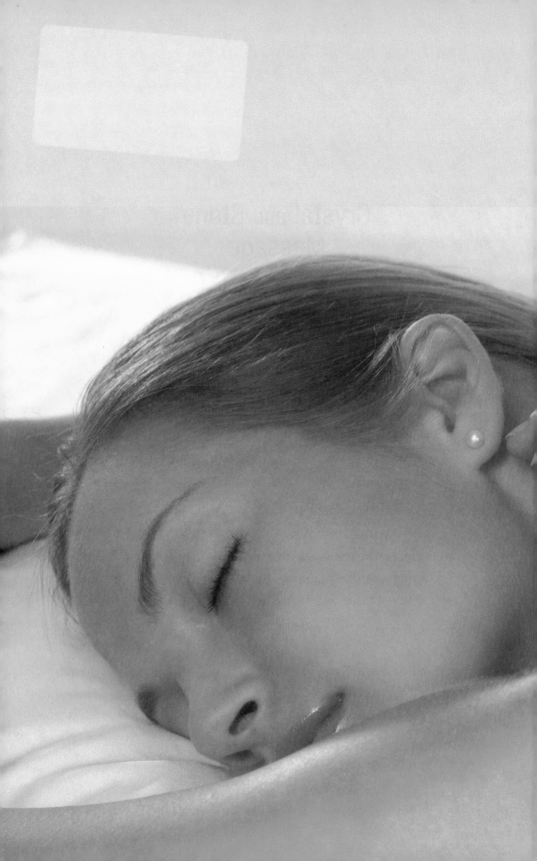

Crystal and Stone Massage

Energy Healing for the Vital and Subtle Bodies

Michael Gienger

with contributions by Hildegard Weiss
and Ursula Dombrowsky

Translated by Tom Blair

Healing Arts Press
Rochester, Vermont • Toronto, Canada

Healing Arts Press
One Park Street
Rochester, Vermont 05767
www.HealingArtsPress.com

Healing Arts Press is a division of Inner Traditions International

Originally published in German in 2004 by Neue Erde GmbH, Saarbruecken, Germany,
    under the title *Edelstein-Massagen*
First English language edition published in 2006 by Earthdancer Books, an imprint of
    Findhorn Press in Scotland, under the title *Crystal Massage for Health and Healing*
First U.S. edition published in 2015 by Healing Arts Press

Note to the reader: *This book is intended as an informational guide. The remedies, approaches,
and techniques described herein are meant to supplement, and not to be a substitute for,
professional medical care or treatment. They should not be used to treat a serious ailment
without prior consultation with a qualified health care professional.*

Library of Congress Cataloging-in-Publication Data
Gienger, Michael.
  [Edelstein-Massagen. English]
  Crystal and stone massage : energy healing for the vital and subtle bodies / Michael
Gienger ; with contributions by Hildegard Weiss and Ursula Dombrowsky ; translated by
Tom Blair . — Second edition.
    pages cm
  Includes index.
  Originally published in German under title: Edelstein-Massagen. Saarbruecken : Neue
Erde, 2014.
  "First English language edition published in 2006 by Earthdancer Books, an imprint
of Findhorn Press in Scotland, under the title Crystal Massage for Health and
Healing"—Preliminaries.
    Summary: "A full-color guide to crystal massage for healing, energy balance, and stress
release in the physical, emotional, and energetic bodies" —Provided by publisher.
  ISBN 978-1-62055-411-1 (paperback) — ISBN 978-1-62055-412-8 (e-book)
  1. Crystals—Therapeutic use. 2. Massage therapy. I. Title.
  RZ415.G54513 2015
  615.8'22—dc23

2014033330

Printed and bound in the United States by Versa Press, Inc.

10 9 8 7 6 5 4 3 2 1

Text design and layout by Virginia Scott Bowman
This book was typeset in Garamond Premier Pro with Helvetica, Futura, and Gill Sans used
    as the display typefaces
Photography by Ines Blersch (www.InesBlersch.de)
Photo models: Michaela Wersebe, Steven Kieltsch

Contents

PART 2

INTUITIVE MASSAGE

PART 3

VITAL BODY MASSAGE

PART 4

HARMONIZING MASSAGE WITH AMBER

By Hildegard Weiss

PART 5

CRYSTAL SPHERE MASSAGE

By Ursula Dombrowsky

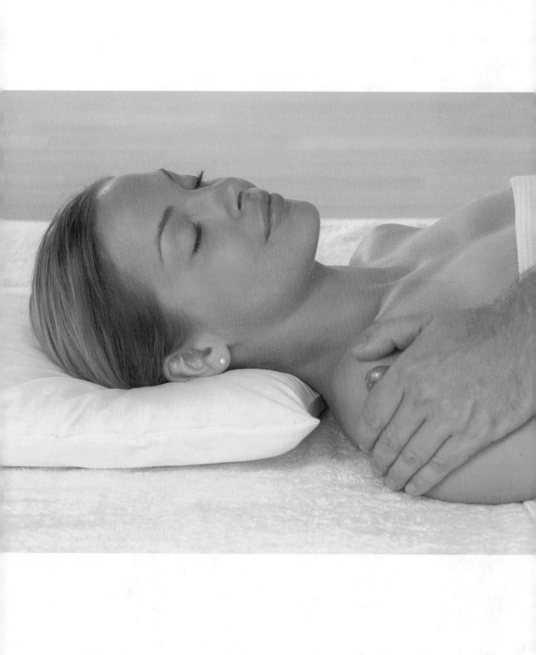

To Touch and Be Touched

To be massaged is surely one of life's most special experiences. Who doesn't enjoy putting oneself in the hands of a trusted masseur or masseuse and allowing nice things to happen? But giving a massage can also be an equally pleasant and transformative experience. To give your focused attention to someone who has put his or her trust in you, and to then see how good your healing touch makes that person feel, is incredibly satisfying.

Massage, from the Arabic *massa,* means "to touch." And deep down, we all long for someone to touch us. This is true in every culture and in every human interaction. Just a glance, a word, or a gesture can touch us. But direct, hands-on contact with another person's body for the purpose of healing is something even more profound. It's too bad that this kind of contact seems to be waning in our world; this may be because we have less time to give or receive massage, because we don't know how to, or because culturally we don't think touching another person other than someone who is very close to us is appropriate.

A world without the kind of physical contact that massage provides would be a much poorer world. By contrast, a world in which human beings touch others in this kind of healing way as a matter of course would be a world rich in empathy, understanding, and compassion.

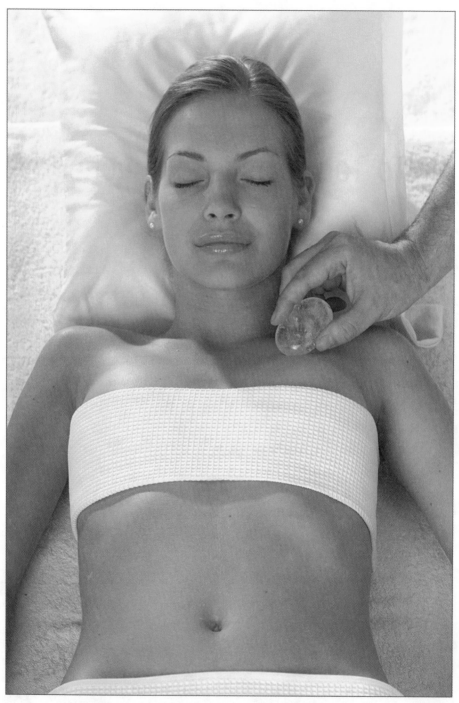

Massage, from the Arabic word *massa*, means "to touch."

For instance, during my time as a shiatsu practitioner I began to notice how much I liked the people I massaged. Regular massages allow our understanding of one another to grow, regardless of any differences in our thinking, behavior, or lifestyle. In the thirteenth-century Icelandic work the *Poetic Edda* we find this: "A gift, and a gift in return, founds friendship, if nothing else opposes it." Could there be any better gift, or gift in return, than to touch another and to be touched?

It's no wonder, then, that massages are so beneficial, and not just for the body, but for the soul, the mind, and the spirit as well. To touch and to be touched always means you are dealing with the whole being; therefore, massage is necessarily holistic healing—as well as a form of healing, by the way, that anyone can give or receive. This is because the essence of healing massage is not technique, but rather the quality of turning to another person with the clear intention of doing good—to provide well-being and healing. If we open ourselves up to this kind of tuning in to others, our hands will usually know what will feel good to the person under them, and what has to be done to achieve this state of well-being. For this reason, I believe that precisely following textbook instructions in massage technique is much less important than *how* we approach the massage, the spirit in which we offer it.

With this book we would like to introduce you to a new dimension of massage, one that incorporates the energetics of crystals and gemstones. Crystals and massage, you may ask? This might seem like a strange or unlikely combination, because most of us tend to think of crystals as being hard or heavy, or containing rough or sharp edges. But you might be surprised to discover how soft crystals and gemstones can actually be, the delicate action they can transmit to the skin and body, and how much light energy they can transmit. Crystal and gemstone massage combines the wonderful advantages of massage, with its intensive tactile contact, with the harmonious, subtle healing bestowed through the luminous energy of the types of stones being used. Depending on how the crystals and stones are applied, we can work on different levels: physical, ethereal, mental, or spiritual. The result is always holistic, and yet each of

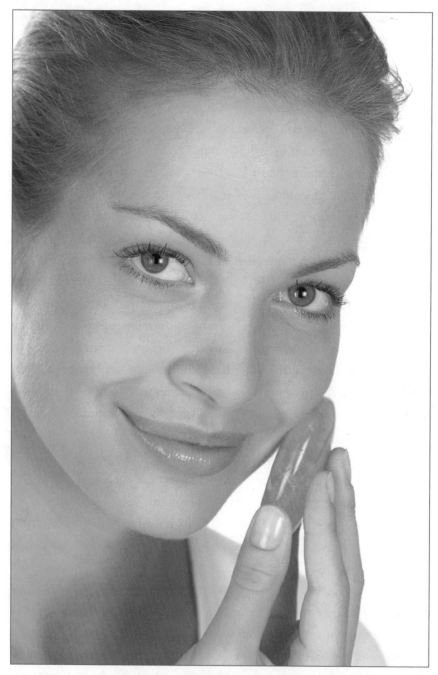

You might be surprised to discover the delicate action crystals and gemstones transmit to the body.

these approaches has a different point of access. Each one opens a different door to us, to our inner world.

This book is divided into five parts and addresses a broad spectrum of readers, from those who have no experience giving massage but who are curious about and interested in—and certainly capable of—using gemstones and crystals in healing bodywork; to experienced massage therapists who want to expand their repertoire of services to their clients and are keen to learn more about how to incorporate crystals and gemstones into their practice. In part 1, "Massage Basics," I walk the reader who may be less experienced in the art of massage through the basic steps of giving a massage.

In part 2, "Intuitive Massage," I focus on how to work with crystals and gemstones, including different techniques, and how some of the different shapes of massage stones can be manipulated to achieve certain effects. Here too I include a list of all the minerals commonly found in crystal massage today and suggest the specific kinds of healing effects that each type of gemstone can provide.

The concept of the vital body is explored in part 3, "Vital Body Massage," where I walk the reader through a whole-body vital massage sequence using crystals.

In the last two parts of this book I present contributions from two esteemed colleagues. In part 4, "Harmonizing Massage with Amber," Hildegard Weiss, an eclectic healer whose work blends crystal massage with her background in craniosacral massage, Bach flower remedies, astrology, and the teachings of Hildegard von Bingen and Thich Nhat Hanh, guides readers through a step-by-step massage sequence using amber, which has a multitude of wonderful healing attributes. And in part 5, "Crystal Sphere Massage," Ursula Dombrowsky, a medical massage therapist who has been incorporating crystals into her work for many years, walks us through a whole-body massage sequence incorporating crystal spheres, a most potent healing tool! My gratitude to both of these contributors, who have been so generous in their willingness to describe these massage techniques they have developed.

I would also like to thank Marco Schreier, a gemstone expert who specializes in the use of stones for health and wellness, who was the initial inspiration for this book and who let us dig deeply into his stock of crystals. I also offer thanks to Sabine Schneider-Kühnle for accompanying the project; to my German publisher, Andreas Lentz, for his willingness to publish this book in its original German edition; to Fred Hageneder for his sure instincts in the design of that edition; to Arwen Lentz for first publishing an English-language translation of this work; and to Tom Blair and Roselle Angwin for their work on that initial translation.

My sincere thanks to my U.S. publisher, Inner Traditions International, and their skillful team of editors for this new edition you hold in your hands.

My gratitude as well to Franca Bauer, Gabriele Simon, Dagmar Fleck, and Erik Frey for providing me with their best massage crystals; and to Ewald Kliegel and my wife, Anja Gienger, for their dedication in performing massage in front of the camera. I would like to thank Eva-Lena Kurtz for assistance in the studio; Steven Kieltsch and Michaela Wersebe for their inspiring contribution as models (especially Michaela, for all of her patience, endurance, and talent); and Stefan Fischer for arranging for me to meet Michaela and Steven. Finally, this book would not be what it is without Ines Blersch's professional eye: she has succeeded in taking really enchanting photos.

I now invite you, the reader, to try out any of the crystal massages that appeal to you that are described in this book, or to come up with your own variations. Whether you are a professional healer interested in integrating crystals as part of your practice or a layperson wanting to make the most of an opportunity for a lovely exchange with a partner, friend, or acquaintance, it is our intention that you find the information contained in this book both practical and inspiring. Our experiences using crystals and stones have been consistently positive:

massage, when combined with the use of crystals and gemstones, can provide us with a more intensive experience of the healing effects of crystals. We believe there is hardly anything more enjoyable than combining the power of touch with the many healing properties of stones.

MICHAEL GIENGER

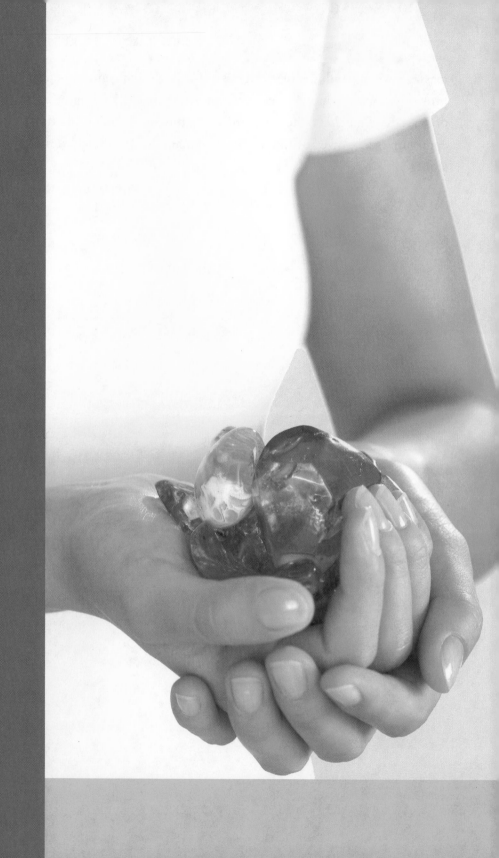

Part 1

Massage Basics

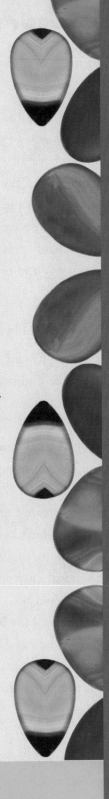

There can be no better gift, or gift in return, than to touch another and to be touched, for by doing so we foster a world rich in empathy, understanding, and compassion.

A MOMENT OF MEETING

A massage is a special moment of meeting. It is therefore very important to devote the proper attention to this moment—enough time to be able to enjoy the massage, and enough time for the massage to continue to have an effect after the session has ended. This means both the amount of time that we are wholeheartedly willing to give to the session and to the person we are working on, and also the amount of time that our counterpart is willing to accept. We have to be willing to be completely present, so that we can direct our undivided attention to the massage and to the person being massaged.

THE PHYSICAL ENVIRONMENT

Having a pleasant and safe space where both parties feel comfortable and will be undisturbed for the duration of the session is vital to a successful experience. This kind of physical environment helps both parties cultivate the "being here now" aspect of massage that creates the feeling of total immersion in the massage, what I refer to as the "inner room." Establishing this kind of environment can compensate for quite a lot if the outer conditions are not ideal. Nevertheless, it is still worthwhile to create a pleasant physical space, because the massage and its effects will be longer lasting and more satisfying.

A comfortably warm, quiet place where you will not be disturbed is the ideal environment for a crystal massage. Warmth is important, as the person who is receiving the massage will usually be unclothed. Some areas of the body may be covered with a blanket during the massage, but for some people any kind of cover can be disturbing, as they want to enjoy total freedom and heightened sensitivity. It is a good idea, therefore, to have a heater of some kind available in case it is needed.

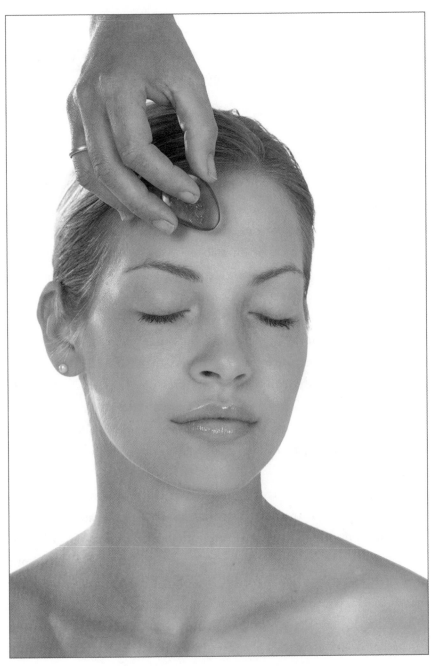

A pleasant and safe space is vital to a
successful massage experience.

A well-designed room with a relaxing atmosphere can help the person receiving the massage to let go, and thus to better receive the massage. A positive response to the ambience of the room sets the stage for successful results.

TREATMENT SURFACE AND CLOTHING

The massage surface can vary, depending on the type of massage being given and the situation. Massage may be administered on the floor, on a firm mattress, or on two or three woolen blankets (such as tightly woven yoga blankets) covered with a sheet, forming a treatment surface. Even better is a massage table, if one is available. Some people can relax better on the floor, as this can provide a more grounded experience. If the massage is being given at home, a bed can be used, but be aware that a mattress that is too soft can affect the massage because it can make direct pressure difficult, as the body gives way, or it can make changing positions difficult because of the lack of resistance. Pillows, knee rolls, woolen blankets, and additional cushions are useful props and should always be within reach during the massage.

I recommend loose-fitting, lightweight clothing, preferably made of natural fibers, for the person giving the massage, because it can get pretty warm during the session. Even though there is not a lot of physical exertion required to give a massage with crystals and stones, your own energy will start flowing strongly—one of the advantages of giving massage. As well, for this reason it is recommended that both parties drink a lot of pure water on the day of the massage (and, of course, go to the bathroom shortly before the massage starts), so that both persons' energy can flow well.

CHOOSING CRYSTALS AND STONES

Rounded semiprecious tumbled stones (i.e., worry stones), crystal massage wands, crystal rods, rounded lens- and soap-shaped stones, and in certain massages even rough stones, crystals, and crystal essences are all appropriate choices for crystal massage.

Crystal massage wands are usually hexagonal, with a rounded base and tip. They should be eight to ten centimeters (approximately three to four inches) in length for best handling. Crystal massage styluses look like elongated teardrops and have a wider base and a thinner, more pointed but slightly rounded tip; these are usually eight to twelve centimeters (about three to four-and-three-quarter inches) long. The wider end has a more relaxing and comforting effect in some techniques, and the more pointed end has a more activating, vitalizing effect.

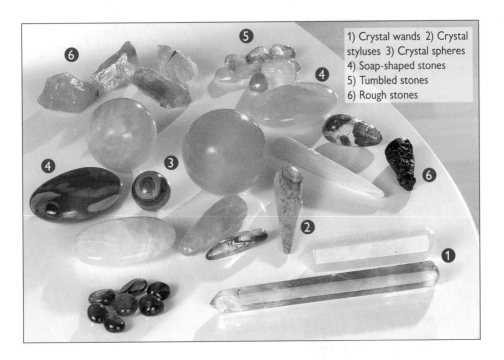

1) Crystal wands 2) Crystal styluses 3) Crystal spheres 4) Soap-shaped stones 5) Tumbled stones 6) Rough stones

Crystal wands and styluses, and the multitude of effects they can produce, are discussed in greater detail in part 3, "Vital Body Massage." As well, the detailed list of the many minerals used in massage, including a discussion of their qualities and healing properties, found in part 2 of this book, provides an excellent overview of the possibilities of healing massage with stones.

Lens-shaped and soap-shaped gemstones, which are flat, oval, polished massage stones, are really ideal for massages, because they have so many application possibilities (unlike tumbled stones, which are unevenly polished pocket stones). Both variations are slightly curved and pleasantly rounded on the edges. Soap-shaped stones are somewhat larger—about the size of a small bar of soap—while lens-shaped stones are somewhat smaller, as seen in the photo below. In principle, basically any stone with a polished surface that doesn't have sharp edges can be used for crystal massages; however, lens- and soap-shaped stones have a multitude of different application possibilities and should be part of any massage stone collection.

For a description of the different effects that can be achieved using "handy" lens- and soap-shaped stones, see part 2, "Intuitive Massage."

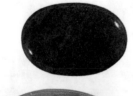

Lens-shaped stone (45 by 35 mm, or approximately 1.75 by 1.5 inches)

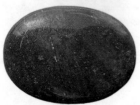

Soap-shaped stone (70 by 50 mm, or approximately 2.75 by 2 inches)

MASSAGE OIL

Massage oil, often used in conventional massage, is usually not needed in crystal massage because the stones' polished surfaces slide well on skin. Furthermore, the effect of some massage techniques in vital body massage, which concentrates on treating the person on the energetic, whole-body level, and not just the physical level, as discussed in part 3, can even be slowed by oil. If you do work with oils you should use high-quality, organic vegetable body oils; good oil can enhance the success of many massages, but low-quality oils slow and block the success.

Things You Need to Give a Crystal Massage

1. A pleasant, safe, quiet space with a good ambience, where you will not be interrupted
2. A treatment surface comfortable for both you and the recipient (a firm mattress, woolen blankets and sheets placed on the floor, or a massage table if available)
3. Comfortable, loose, lightweight clothing
4. Ambient warmth (use a heater if necessary)
5. Pillows, knee rolls, and other such aids for comfort
6. Blanket or sheet to cover the recipient (optional)
7. Tumbled stones, round stones, crystal rods, crystal wands, lens- and soap-shaped stones
8. Massage oil (optional, depending on type of massage)

THE "INNER ROOM"

Before starting the massage, allow yourself and the person whom you are going to massage a few minutes to settle in preparation for the session. For example, a short conversation, perhaps over a glass of water or a cup of tea (followed by a quick bathroom break), and you'll both find yourselves present in a totally different way than if you were to immediately jump onto the massage table or mat, especially directly after a car journey. See that the person receiving the massage is completely comfortable on the treatment surface at the beginning of the massage; use pillows, blanket rolls, or other aids as needed, then cover her with a blanket or sheet, if necessary. Then allow your counterpart (and yourself) a moment or two of peaceful quietude before you begin the session.

Visualize that you are totally present for your counterpart during this time. Everything else must be secondary when you give a massage—your everyday life, your problems, your interests, and yes, even your own well-being. Consciously put it all aside, knowing you can return to your concerns afterward, and direct all your attention to the massage.

> It is not only your hands that function while giving a massage; it is also your mind, your feelings, and your perceptions. Therefore, prepare yourself by allowing your mind to settle and become quiet, neutral, and focused on the well-being of your client or partner.

CREATING PROTECTION

Before you begin your work, create a protective psychic boundary around yourself, wherein everything that belongs to you stays with you, and everything that belongs to your counterpart stays with her or him. "Foreign" energy, the psychic energy that belongs to another, is always a weight, especially when you are doing bodywork of any kind, where psychic sensitivity is heightened. The goal of a massage is to dissolve another person's tension and blocks, and to do this you must let your own energy flow unimpeded.

> Flowing energy is available energy. Energy that does not flow is bound, blocked, or trapped in some way. We each have our own vital energy, in sufficient amounts that we don't need the energy of another. We each live by our own efforts.

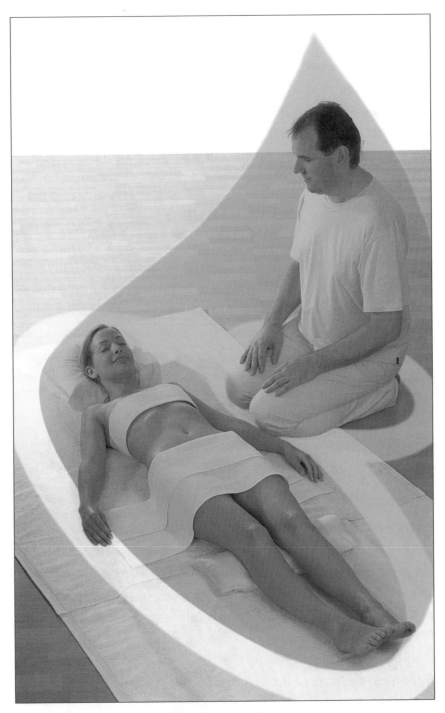

Creating protection

You can create such a safe environment by first determining that everything stays where it should, or returns to where it comes from. You can then visualize a violet light around your counterpart and yourself as a horizontal figure eight—two circles that touch but still separately enclose each of you. But whether you use this visualization or another one to create a protective boundary, the most important thing is that you and the person you are massaging are always safe.

CULTIVATING INTUITION

Protected as you now are, begin to consciously cultivate your intuition in order to tune in to the needs of the person you are massaging. Intuition is the "sixth sense," after the five ordinary senses of sight, hearing, smell, touch, and taste. While massaging, we are especially dependent on this sense, as it allows us to sense, not from the mind, but from the heart, how a person is feeling and what they are needing. A massage is especially good if you can work intuitively instead of simply technically, as one's intuition can guide one's hands during the session.

Using crystals and stones in an intuitive way in massage is discussed in greater detail in the next part of this book, "Intuitive Massage."

Intuition can run both ways during a treatment, in that both the giver of the massage and the receiver can synchronize, attuning to the same wavelength. One way of doing this is to begin to inhale and exhale fully and completely, asking your counterpart or client to bring his attention to his breath and follow your breathing like this for a few minutes (people who are tense will often breathe in short, shallow, or interrupted breaths). By synchronizing your breathing in this way at the start of the massage, you can pick up on your client's energy, while your client can begin to tune in to the massage energy you are sending out. If you've never tried this before, it may feel unusual, but once you try it out a few times you will soon see that it helps give you a pretty good sense of what is good for the person you are massaging, and that sense of inner knowing about what the person needs will remain throughout the session even as you each return to your normal breathing rhythms.

First Steps:
Preparing for the Crystal Massage

1. Identify a comfortable position for the person being treated, using such aids as pillows or towel rolls, as needed.
2. Settle your mind, allow extraneous concerns to drop away, and focus your awareness solely on the massage.
3. Create a protective boundary, knowing that everything stays where it should, or returns to where it comes from. Use the violet light, figure-eight visualization, or some other form of protection you are familiar with.
4. Cultivate your intuition in order to tune in empathically to the person being massaged. Use the synchronized breathing exercise or some other technique to establish mutual attunement.

POSTURE AND POSITION

Your position during the massage will be determined by the treatment surface you are using, whether it is the floor or a massage table. In either case it is important that you be in a comfortable position, in which you can straighten up and lean forward without strain. The right sitting or kneeling position is important while working on the floor, while the correct height adjustment is important if you are standing and using a massage table. It is always advantageous to begin in a centered position, so that throughout the massage you can always return to your own center. And always check at the beginning of the massage that you are in a position that you can sustain comfortably over an extended period of time. Some massage positions are unusual, but many things can be rectified by a small correction of your posture or position; this conserves a lot of energy.

Posture and position are discussed in greater detail in subsequent parts of this book that pertain to the various types of crystal massage.

USING THE WHOLE BODY AND THE BREATH

Whichever massage techniques are employed—grips, movements, and application of the crystals—will depend on which crystal massage you have chosen to do and the specific area of the body being massaged. In general, though, any technique you are using will be less strenuous if you engage your whole body. And so whether you are doing small, fine movements, such as those used in vital body massage, as described in detail in part 3 of this book, or whether you are using more pressure, as in a massage with crystal spheres, described by Ursula Dombrowsky in part 5, it is always more efficient and less taxing to let your movements be generated by your *entire* body, using gravity to assist you as you lean in and out.

Here I suggest a little exercise. Sit in front of a table, and push against the edge of the table with both thumbs. First do it with the strength of the muscles in your arms. The movement will be relatively jerky, and you will feel this through your whole body. No notable energy flow develops, and soon it starts to be strenuous. Now push your thumbs against the edge of the table by shifting your entire body back and forth. Your arm muscles merely hold, but do not do the actual pushing. In this way you will find that the movements are much more harmonious, the pressure changes more fluidly, and a flow of energy develops within you, with the overall result that it is hardly strenuous at all. Can you feel the difference?

This principle is not only true in massage, as moving in this way prevents fatigue, tension, pain, injury, and other ailments in many

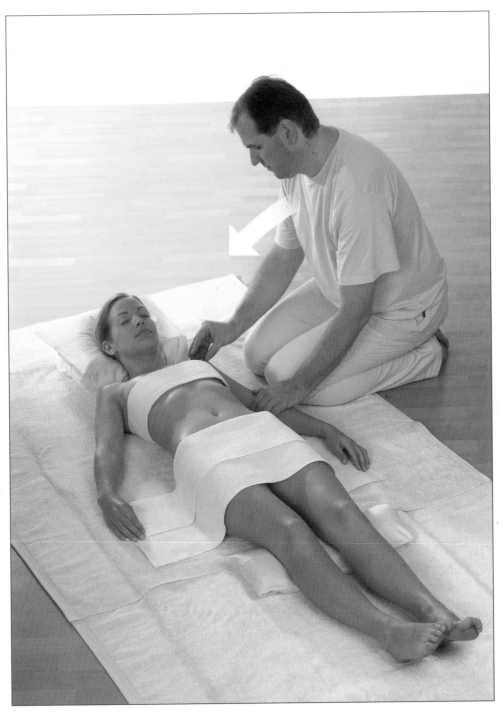

Engage your whole body while working.

different types of activities, from opening a tight jar lid to engaging in different kinds of sports. It is even better if you synchronize your physical movements with your breath. So for example, when you perform a massage technique that requires effort, such as pushing, gripping, or lifting, do it on an exhalation; this allows you to conserve your energy, and it will also feel more pleasant. You then release or pause in your movement on an inhalation. This precise delineation might not be possible with all massage techniques, but where the rhythm of exertion and letting go exists (no matter how subtle), this breathing pattern can be very helpful in terms of conserving your energy. Once you are accustomed to working this way, you will find it comes quite naturally and you'll begin to use your breath like this even in everyday, commonplace activities. For example, I cured my chronic backaches during my time as a paramedic by using this simple technique.

NONVERBAL FEEDBACK AND RELEASES

If you are massaging for the first time you may need to remind yourself to pay attention to the various forms of feedback from the person as you massage. Simply remember to regularly direct your attention to the well-being of the person you are working on and note his or her response. Facial expression, breathing, involuntary movements, bowel sounds (often a sign of relaxation), and vocal utterances all provide feedback. This feedback is very important in making sure you are on the right track. And if you are a professional massage therapist you know that the better your command of the various massage techniques, the more your attention will be freed for this kind of observation.

Note that the danger of any routine—particularly if you are a more seasoned massage therapist—is that we don't stay present, and our minds tend to wander. If this is the case, then you're just massaging technically, by rote, while being absent spiritually. In this case the massage will not be deeply effective, even though you may be doing everything correctly from a technical standpoint. But what's missing is presence, atmosphere, spirit.

If you catch your mind wandering, even having this awareness is an important first step. Give yourself a quick reminder of the need at all times to be totally present, to devote yourself entirely to the massage, and return your full attention to the person under your hands.

Be prepared for releases. Massages loosen things up, and anything that loosens stuck energy initiates a reaction. It is reassuring, of course, when relaxation and well-being result from a massage, but sometimes something that stands in the way of balance and lasting well-being has to be released in the person being massaged. So don't be afraid if a client moans or sighs, and especially if they cry. These are all healthy responses to the release of bound-up energy, particularly if the energy has been stuck for a long time. Know that massages that produce these kinds of reactions often bring the most relief. If you notice tense facial

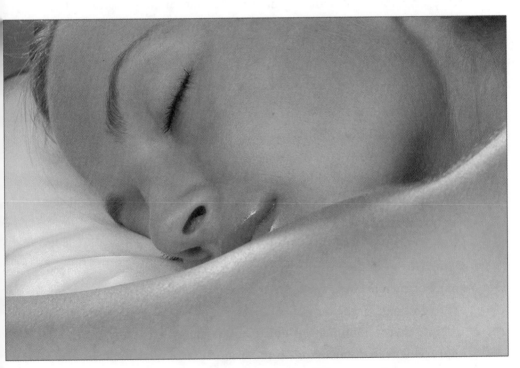

Pay attention to feedback, however obvious or subtle.

expressions or sounds of discomfort, don't hesitate to ask what's going on. Some things just have to be expressed before they can be resolved. If tears begin to flow, ask if you should pause or if you should continue, and reassure the person that this kind of response is normal and perfectly fine within the context of the healing brought on by the massage. Give her permission to vocalize or cry. Don't interrupt this kind of release by assuming the person needs consoling. Just remain present and empathic, whether continuing to massage or pausing, and allow the tears to flow. As you know, a good cry can sometimes feel so good.

If you have paused during such a release, just wait until the tears have stopped flowing (and offer tissues if needed), and then continue with the massage. Certainly do not stop at this point, if at all possible—tears are a sign that the massage is doing its work. You can always be assured that sunshine follows the rain, bringing newfound clarity and energy. It's important that you conclude the massage on an uplift, which will definitely arrive if you continue to massage thoroughly, gently, and sensitively, always being totally there for your client.

END ON THE UPLIFT

Notice the turning point in the massage, when an uplift in the person's energy occurs. This moment of uplift often comes toward the end of the massage but may occur before the planned conclusion. Suddenly the person beneath your hands will breathe a sigh of relief, smile joyfully, maybe even start to laugh, or otherwise look blissful. Does it get any better than this? Hardly! So the best thing to do once you notice this is to plan to wind down at this point. Finish the area you are massaging (for example, finish the second leg if you have only massaged one), but then begin to work toward a conclusion. You want the recipient to go home in the best possible state.

Note that the moment of uplift can be identified as any *noticeable* improvement in comparison to the original state of the person when she arrived at the session. This is not necessarily an outright expression of bliss; sometimes, especially if we are new to massage, we can only accomplish small steps with a massage. But every improvement, however small or large, should be considered a sign of success.

If you happen to work past this high point, if the glow disappears and the emotions of your partner seem to sink, you can ask for feedback—"Where was it best?"—after you have completed the area you are working on. The recollection alone is sometimes enough to let the feeling return to the person. If not, just ask, "Should I go back to that place?" If the answer is yes, a brief return to the area that produced the moment of uplift is usually sufficient to restore the person's positive response. If the client indicates that you should continue, then simply go on with the massage, knowing that you will always find a way to the uplift, provided you stay in touch with your intuition and remain present, focused on the person's well-being.

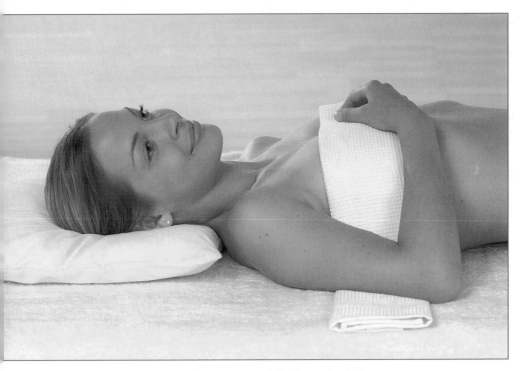

Conclude on an "uplift," often signaled
by a sigh of relief or a joyful smile.

Massage Reminders

1. Find a comfortable position for yourself from which you can massage from your center.
2. Engage your whole body, and let gravity work for you as you synchronize your breathing with your movements.
3. Keep your attention solely on the massage and the person you are massaging, and return to that point of focus if your attention wanders.
4. Allow releases that herald relief to arise uninterrupted. Give your client the necessary time and space to release energy blocks and then continue with the massage; don't suffocate tears with over-hasty consolation—tears are a positive response.
5. Conclude the massage at the moment of uplift.

When the massage ends, it is sometimes best to stay in the room (both physically and spiritually) for a few moments, quietly observing the energy of the person you have just worked on. Just stay seated close by. Use your intuition, and be responsive to whatever is needed in the situation, whether it is simply a silent presence or the person would like to talk about the massage. Give the person the space she needs, and withdraw if that's what's appropriate. You can say, "Take the time you need, and get up when you're ready," if you decide to leave the room. You have then communicated that there is enough time to allow the effects of the massage to settle, as much time as is desired.

DISSOLVING THE PROTECTIVE ENVELOPE AND CLEARING LINGERING ENERGY

At this point you might want to remind yourself that everything that belongs to you stays with you, and that everything that belongs to the person you have just massaged stays with her. You might envisage this as a short-term connection, during which an exchange of energy has taken place; dissolve the violet light of protection that you established at the start of the session as the massage ends. Interestingly enough, you may notice relief in yourself as well as in your partner. This confirms that it was indeed a beneficial exchange for both parties.

If you sense that something is still lingering in the space between you and your partner following the massage, it could be some residual energy—beliefs, ideas, emotions, and so on—that belong to the person you have just worked on. In such a case, you can use the following clearing technique to clear the room, yourself, or the larger space around you and your counterpart:

Picture this energy as consisting of many small particles, then direct the following silent command purposefully toward the particles: *Return to the moment of your creation—or be free!* You might have to send this thought out a few times, but you will soon recognize that what was left in the room has dissolved and disappeared. When doing this kind of clearing, it's helpful to remember that energy is simply energy, neither "bad" nor "good," and that it is best for all things to be in their right place; i.e., free.

This final clearing and dissolving of absorbed and unwanted energy is a great help to you, so that you are not weighed down with someone else's energetic ballast. It is equally helpful to your counterpart, who might not be aware that the energy she most likely just unloaded during this session lingers. In addition to this clearing, if you like you can also clear your massage space with resonance spheres or bowls or tuning forks, or by burning some sage or incense; they all work in the same way. And this kind of clearing, if done while the person you have massaged is still present, can make for a wonderful conclusion for both of you.

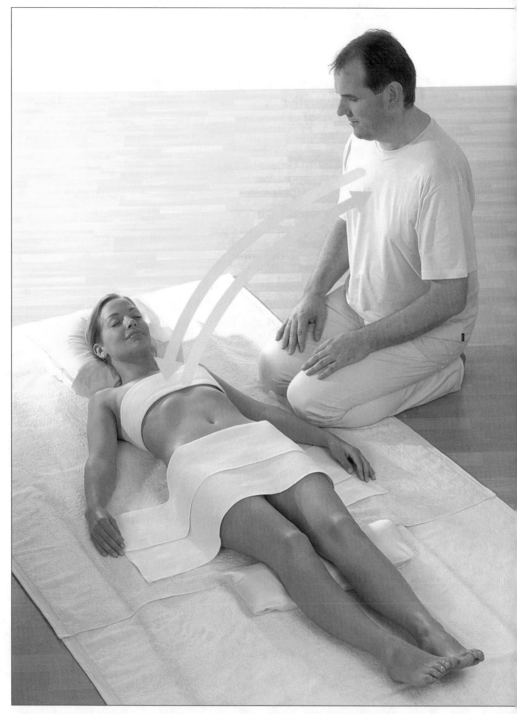

Dissolve the protective envelope at the conclusion of the session.

GETTING FEEDBACK

Following the massage, any kind of feedback you get from your partner about the effects can be quite illuminating and rewarding, as every massage session is an opportunity to learn more and to sharpen your senses and skills. You can check to see if the person's report corresponds to your own observations; sharing this kind of information can be beneficial for both parties. However, only seek feedback right after a session *if the person so desires to give it to you*. If you've never worked with crystals in this way before, it's sometimes tempting to fish around for feedback, but forcing a conversation at this point can undermine the success of the session; let your counterpart initiate any dialogue. As well, very often perceptions of the effects of a crystal massage only come into one's consciousness some time afterward, as it gently continues to have positive effects; therefore it is sometimes advantageous to wait for feedback to arise naturally.

Once the massage has ended and the person has departed, you can

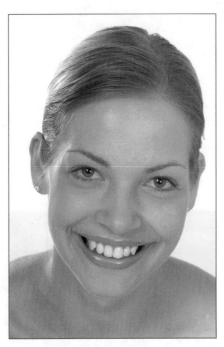

The effects of crystal massages are lasting.

slip out of your role as therapist. What you set aside before the session may now be taken back, if you (still) want to. It is also good to leave the treatment room, at least for a short break, but to then tidy it, to return it to its previous state, before the massage.

CLEANSING THE CRYSTALS

Finally, you should be sure to cleanse the crystals and stones you used during the session of any absorbed energy and information. Hold them under

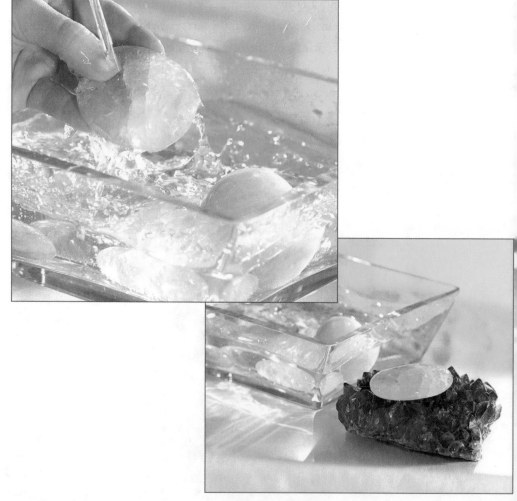

Cleansing the crystals

running water for a minute or longer, and rub them vigorously with your fingers. As you do this, you will notice that the surface of the stones feels somewhat soapy in the beginning, and then a resistance will start to build, until after a while the rubbing finger will not slide anymore. That shows you that any absorbed energy has been washed away. Take the crystals out of the water, and lay them on an amethyst geode or a piece of an amethyst geode. The amethyst will free the stones of the last of the "foreign" information and restore them to a pristine state. After a few hours of amethyst cleansing, your crystal will be ready for your next treatment.

Concluding the Massage

1. In a very "present" way, observe and ask about the well-being of your counterpart. Be sure to leave time for any needs that may follow.

2. Dissolve the energetic protective envelope you created earlier, and clear any remaining energy stuck in the room with the silent command, *Return to the moment of your creation—or be free!*

3. Discuss the effects of the massage, but only if the person indicates such a conversation is desired.

4. Consciously release your therapist role, and return to your everyday life. If necessary, leave the room, or you can tidy it up following the session.

5. Cleanse your crystals and stones under flowing water, and place on an amethyst geode.

The basic steps described in this chapter are performed in all the crystal massages outlined in this book. Some massage techniques deemphasize certain steps, whereas others emphasize them. This is the nature of the work. It is very helpful to memorize the fundamentals found in this chapter, or to write them down as crib notes. But don't simply copy the summaries provided throughout this chapter; find a way to make notes that are meaningful to you personally. Once you've noted the steps, perhaps using meaningful key words, you'll tend to remember the steps better later, as needed.

LAST WORDS

Please, do yourself and the other person a favor: do not give a crystal massage if you are unfit or unwell, or are not in a good mood. As mentioned before, it is not only your hands that affect the massage, but also your moods and thoughts, and crystals are very sensitive to the vibrations of our emotions. If the timing is not right for you, the effects for both parties will not be satisfying. You should always be able to keep a neutral mind-set for crystal massage work, just observing and doing what is best for your client. Therefore, do not let yourself be persuaded to give a massage if you are not willing to or if the basic conditions are not right (the possible indications and contraindications of the different types of crystal massage described later in this book are mentioned in the relevant chapters).

On the other hand, if you feel fit and wide awake, if there are no basic concerns and you would enjoy giving a massage, you will be able to achieve wonderful results. The range of possible benefits is huge. We can relieve tired muscles, bones and joints can be made fit, and we can positively impact a multitude of other ailments, moods, and mental conditions, too. You will find out more about this in subsequent chapters.

> The crystal massages mentioned in this book serve primarily as ways to achieve well-being and to mobilize self-healing forces. They have been proven and tested in practice but are naturally not a substitute for diagnoses or treatments from doctors or alternative practitioners. You should always ask for competent advice if confronted with a serious condition, and only administer a crystal massage after consulting the treating specialists.

In the end, you learn to massage by massaging. Everything else develops accordingly. Crystal massage is an art that has to be practiced and experienced. But the rewarding thing about crystal massage

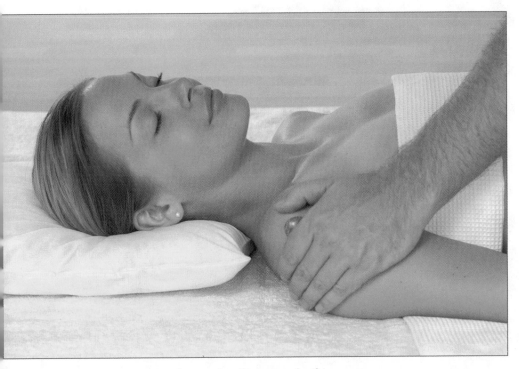

Just trying it out can be fun.

is that it can be fun and healing for both parties, bringing happiness and well-being. As German poet and satirist Erich Kästner once said, "There is no good unless you do it." This is especially true in massage. That being said, let's explore the possibilities . . .

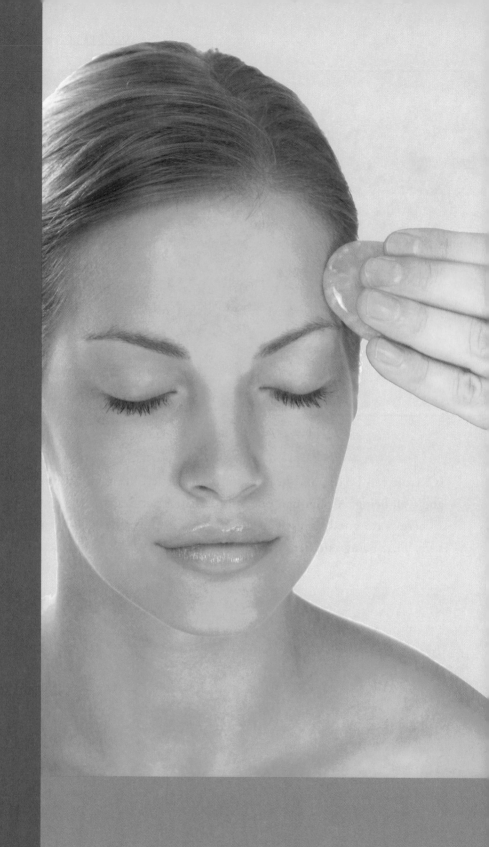

Part 2

Intuitive Massage

■

Intuition is the "sixth sense," after the five ordinary senses of sight, hearing, smell, touch, and taste. While massaging, we are especially dependent on this sense, as it allows us to sense, not from the mind, but from the heart, how a person is feeling and what he is needing.

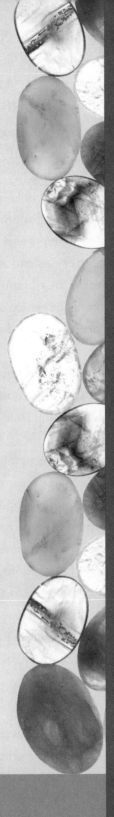

ACQUIRING KNOWLEDGE
THROUGH INNER PERCEPTION

Great news: massaging another person feels good! What's more, success is almost certain if we proceed carefully and sensitively, if we observe the results of what we are doing closely, and most of all, if we rely on our intuition to guide our hands. As discussed in part 1 (and as attested to by most professional massage therapists), intuition, our "sixth sense," is far more important in massage work than technique. This is particularly true in crystal and stone massage, as crystals and gemstones are extremely sensitive to vibration and carry their own distinct healing energies that can only be sensed and conveyed through the hands of a massage practitioner who is comfortable relying on inner perception.

You only need a few round, polished crystals and some basic experience in the various massage steps, as described in the previous chapter. Pay particular attention to the first steps of settling your mind and synchronizing your breathing; this will facilitate your tuning in to your intuition.

If you are new to the use of gemstones and crystals in massage, it will be helpful to try out the different massage techniques outlined in this part of the book by first practicing mini-massages on yourself, on different areas of your body. In this way you'll gain firsthand experience in the use of crystals and stones, and you'll come to know the possibilities and limitations of the different applications so that you can apply these correctly to others. Once you have experienced, at least once, how various massage techniques feel, the appropriate movements will come much more naturally and unerringly when you massage others.

So now, let's go!

MASSAGE TECHNIQUES

Try each of the techniques below, making movements with the crystal or stone on the skin of your inner forearm, your chest and abdomen, or on your thigh—anyplace where you can massage yourself effectively and comfortably, observing the results and allowing them to shape your inner perception.

Begin by holding the stone in your hand firmly but not in such a way as to feel cramping or tension while massaging. You should have the feeling that you have the stone safely under control. The security or insecurity by which you hold the stones is transmitted to the person being massaged through the sensitivity of the crystals. Don't grip them, and don't handle them too casually either; such casualness can be misinterpreted by the crystal or the stone as being neglectful. Experiment with this idea using a partner.

Circling: Move the crystal across the skin in circular motions, applying more and less pressure alternately. Try out the differences between small and large circles and different speeds, as well as the difference between the flat surfaces and the rounded edges of the crystal.

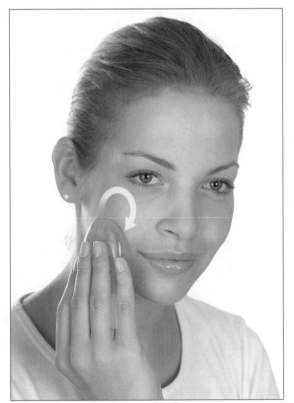

Circling

Rubbing: Guide the stone over the skin in long, straight movements, putting pressure on the surface evenly. Differences result from variation of pressure, speed, and the area being massaged.

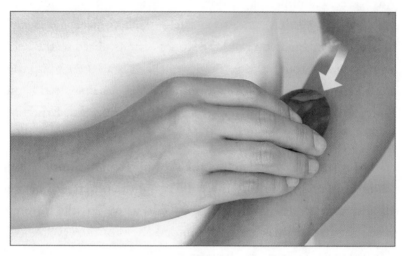

Rubbing

Pulling: Pulling is similar to rubbing, except that it is applied to smaller areas, and more pressure is put onto the back end of the stone (in relation to the direction of movement). As with the other techniques, try varying pressure and speed.

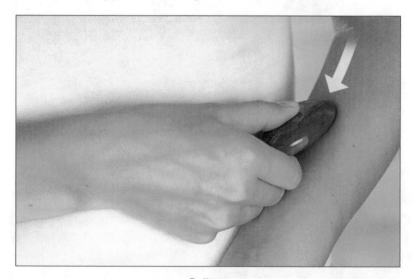

Pulling

Joggle: Moving the crystal back and forth dynamically while rubbing or pulling firmly joggles body parts and muscles. This is a strong loosening movement that needs a certain pressure and speed, but must not be too firm.

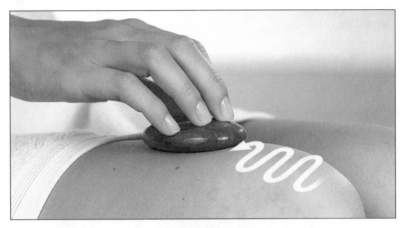

Joggling

Vibrating: The stone is moved up and down dynamically while rubbing or pulling, so that the muscles and body parts vibrate over a large area. You may also vibrate in just one spot for a short time. Experiment to find out what amount of pressure and speed is the most agreeable.

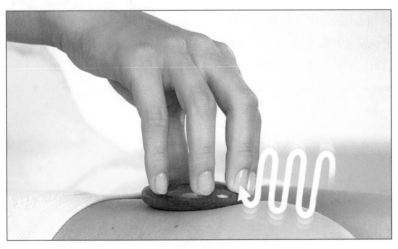

Vibrating

Kneading: Muscles and tissue are worked over with firm pressure and with turning movements of the stone. Try out the minimum pressure and the maximum comfortable edge.

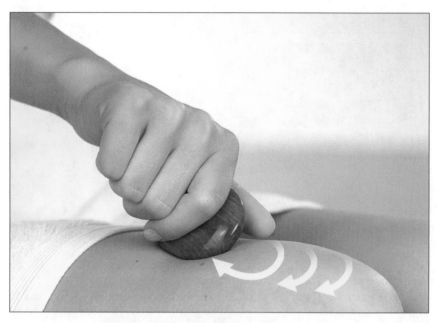

Kneading

Pressing: The crystal is pressed into the muscles briefly, then released, as in pressure-point massage. A line of several pressure points is formed this way. Pressing is an enjoyable and simultaneously deeply loosening technique. It is very important not to apply pressure using muscle power while massaging someone, but only by shifting your own weight (see the previous chapter on basics).

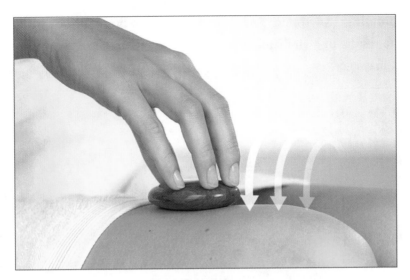

Pressing

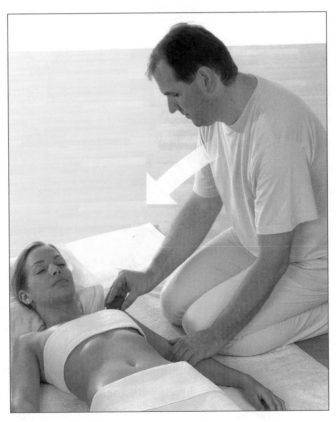

Shift your weight!

Drumming: Rhythmic, soft drumming of the body surface with the stone results in a vitalizing effect. Try to vary the speed, strength, and area massaged.

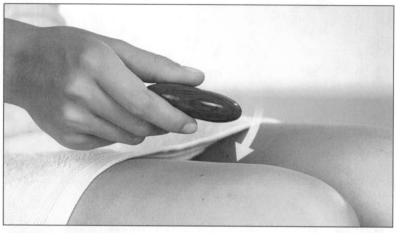

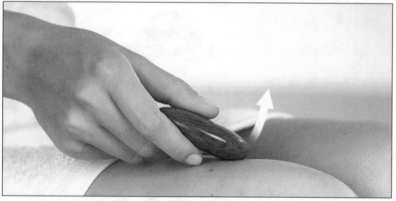

Drumming

There are any number of variations on massage using a healing crystal or gemstone. The techniques described above are fundamental but are not all inclusive, by any means; with intuition and some creativity you can develop additional ideas yourself. After you've experimented on yourself, try out various techniques on a partner, taking turns at massaging as you familiarize yourself with them. Once you have developed a feeling for the basic techniques, the right ones will occur to you at the right moment during an intuitive massage.

CREATING
DIFFERENT EFFECTS

Lens- and soap-shaped gemstones and crystals, described in part 1, are ideal for use by those who have never used stones and crystals before in massage. Not only are they easier for the practitioner to hold and manipulate, the softly rounded edges and flatness of the stones feel wonderful to the recipient of the massage. When you are first experimenting with stones, I recommend these "handy," easily manipulated shapes. The following are some of the many different effects that can be achieved with such stones.

Harmonizing: Firm motions with the flat side of a soap-shaped stone (circling, pulling, kneading, or pressing) on the skin have a harmonizing effect. Hold the stone on its edge or by placing your entire hand on its surface so you can guide it and vary the pressure.

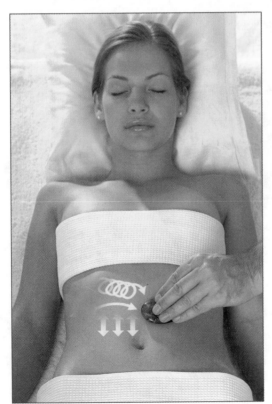

Harmonizing

Stimulating: Motions on the skin with the narrow, i.e., more rounded, edge of the stone are stimulating. This application is very invigorating even if you rub, circle, or pull with just a little pressure. Hold the stone securely to do this.

Energizing: Joggling and vibrating with soap-shaped stones has an energizing effect—an even more stimulating effect. It is advisable to use the flat side of the stone because the edges might feel too intense, though this is not always the case with each person.

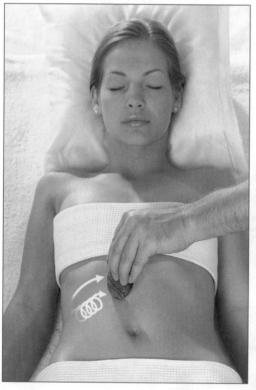

Stimulating

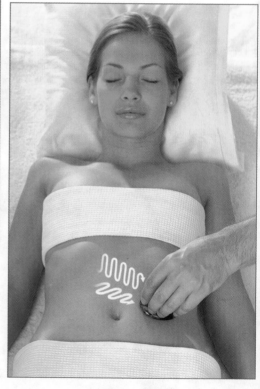

Energizing

Soothing rubbing: Rubbing with the flat side of the soap-shaped stone always offers a relaxing and soothing element during a massage, especially at the conclusion. The stone is held more loosely in this case and placed on the body more gently.

Vitalizing rubbing: Rubbing with the wide side of the stone also has a relaxing effect but is simultaneously vitalizing. It awakens and stimulates and is good at the conclusion of the massage if you want your client to go back into everyday life on an animated note.

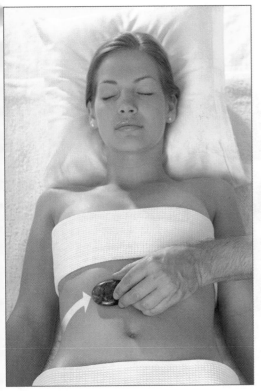

Soothing rubbing

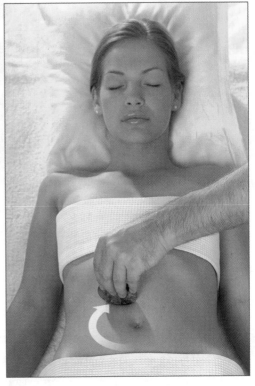

Vitalizing rubbing

THE DIFFERENT STONE AND
CRYSTAL SHAPES

Lens- and soap-shaped gemstones and crystals are only some of the shapes that are used in crystal and stone massage. You have many other choices. Tumbled and polished stones, smooth raw stones, or other shapes, including crystals with defined edges, can be quite effective in a massage. Irregularly shaped stones in particular have peculiarities that are worth exploring. As time goes by, you will be able to assemble your special personal set out of various healing stones and crystals for massage.

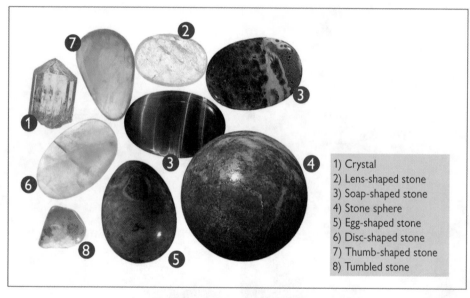

1) Crystal
2) Lens-shaped stone
3) Soap-shaped stone
4) Stone sphere
5) Egg-shaped stone
6) Disc-shaped stone
7) Thumb-shaped stone
8) Tumbled stone

A selection of the various shapes used
in stone and crystal massage

A WHOLE-BODY INTUITIVE
CRYSTAL MASSAGE SEQUENCE

First, lay out the stones and/or crystals you feel will be suitable for carrying out the massage. Let your massage partner find a comfortable position, and determine the parts of the body you are going to focus on. (In practicing, it is sometimes best to massage back and limbs first.) Next, prepare yourself for the massage in the ways outlined in the "first steps" instructions found in part 1, by settling your mind and synchronizing your breathing, so you can tune in to the person you are massaging.

Part 3, "Vital Body Massage," includes a discussion of the effects that can be achieved with a crystal stylus, and a list of the various crystals and stones available in stylus shape. As well, Ursula Dombrowsky's discussion of massage using crystal spheres, found in part 5 of this book, offers guidance on selecting spheres for massage, as well as a list of the most common crystals and stones available in sphere shape.

Then I suggest you just let the massage happen. See where your impulses lead you. Are the shoulders crying out for relaxation? Is it the abdomen that hurts? Are the legs or feet tired? Sometimes you have the sense that you know exactly where to start, and if so, follow this feeling. Otherwise, just begin with the back—this almost always feels good.

In focusing on a certain area, select the stone that jumps to your attention. This will be the stone that your eyes fix on, the stone you just know/see/feel will be right. Make contact with a certain area by first letting your hand rest there with the stone, then follow with the motion that seems to happen by itself, or that is the easiest to carry out. This can be gentle circling, rubbing, pulling, joggling, vibrating, kneading, drumming, or whatever motion seems to be right. Basically, any movement is correct in an intuitive healing massage using gemstones and crystals if you feel that it fits, and if it makes your partner feel good (in my experience, though, pulling motions are usually more pleasant than pushing ones).

Now, massage the entire area using alternating techniques, in any way that feels right. Always observe the reactions of your partner

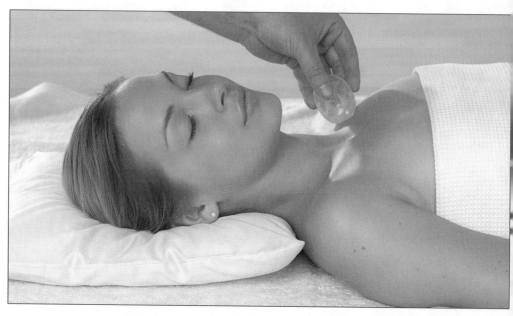

Begin contact by resting the stone on the body.

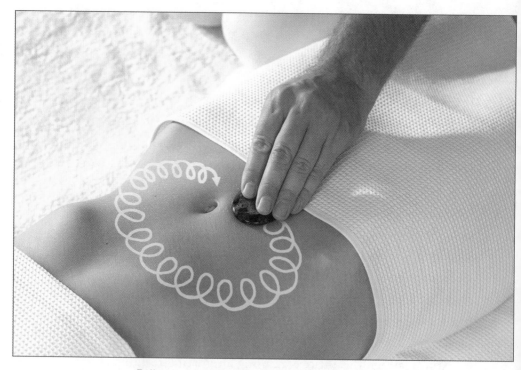

Follow with the motion that comes naturally,
such as gentle circling.

while massaging. Tense muscles may hurt and need a certain amount of pressure to be loosened, so always make sure to alternate relaxing movements with firmer massaging. Alternating between firmness and gentleness makes a crystal massage dynamic and vivid. The aim is to create a pleasant and harmonious action that is neither too limp nor too forceful. This produces results that are the foundation of a healthy feeling that permeates all the way through to the subtle, energetic, vital body.

> Be sure to bring some variety into the massage. The state we are hoping to achieve with the massage is similar to that of a cat crouching: the state of tension in every muscle is related to a deep peace that can last for hours but is still capable of reacting as fast as lightning. Cats are teachers of litheness!

As you move along, massage area by area: for example, the back, the back of the legs and the soles of the feet are one area; the arms another; the chest, abdomen, pelvis, and front of legs compose another area; and finally the head. This way of proceeding section by section allows you to become more familiar with massaging the whole body, and you can then learn to approach the more sensitive areas gradually. It is usually best for the back, legs, and feet if you massage them from top to bottom. This relaxes and dissolves pain. If someone's body is very untoned, though, exactly the opposite direction might be helpful, so follow your intuition and observe what is needed. Massaging the arms is similar to massaging the back and legs: it is usually more enjoyable if you work from top to bottom, from the shoulders to the hands—but this rule is not without its exceptions, either.

Downward and outward motions that follow the course of the ribs are recommended for the chest. Gentle techniques applied clockwise (from the recipient's right side to left side) are best for the abdomen; this direction follows the course of the intestines. Rubbing motions are

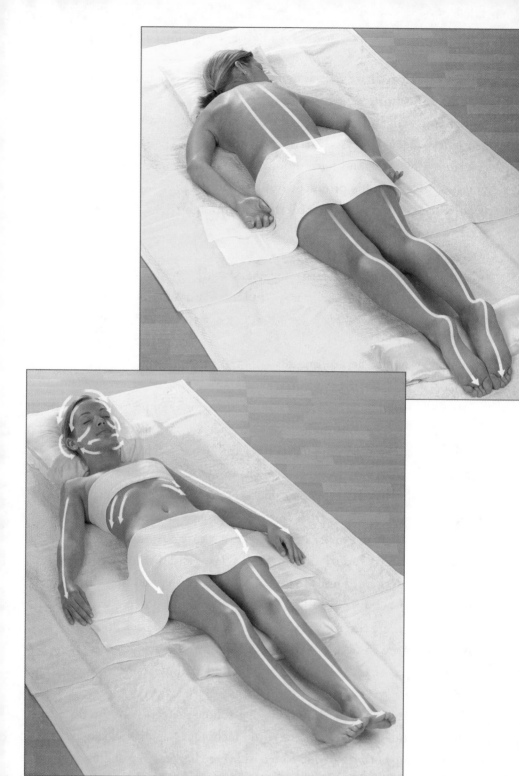

Sequence of a whole-body massage

usually very pleasant for the skull and the nape of the neck. Gentle circling, kneading, or pushing motions, alternating with outward rubbing movements, are good for the face.

Sequence of an Intuitive Stone Massage

1. Lay out the crystals and stones you will use and follow the basic steps to prepare yourself to give a massage (see part 1, "Massage Basics").

2. In focusing on a certain area, select the crystal or stone that seems to immediately draw your attention.

3. Try different massage techniques (e.g., circling, pulling, pressing, rubbing), and vary them; alternate firmness and gentleness, always observing the results.

4. Massage area by area: the back, the back of the legs and soles of the feet; the arms; the chest, abdomen, pelvis, and front of legs; and lastly the head.

5. In general, massage from top to bottom of an area (though there may be exceptions to this rule); downward and outward for the chest; circular and clockwise for the abdomen; and back and forth for the head and neck.

The suggestions given here for the sequence of an intuitive stone massage are only tips, guidance for giving the massage for the first time. However, there are no set rules in intuitive massage. Certainly the more comfortable you are with using your intuition, the more you can rely on it to guide you when giving a massage, even if what you're doing seems to go against all the standard "rules."

It is not necessary, of course, to massage the entire body. Less is often more, especially in the beginning, when you are still learning. Don't strain yourself; only massage for as long as you have enough power, stamina, and attention to do so comfortably. If you notice that you are losing concentration or are getting tense or that your energy is flagging, then finish the massage in the area you are working on and then conclude the session. It is important, though, that you always complete the entire area you have begun. And so if you have massaged one side of the body, massage the corresponding opposite side, too, and always complete both legs or both arms. If you were to leave an area unfinished, a disturbing or unpleasant feeling of imbalance can remain.

Concluding the massage on an uplift, as described in part 1, is ideal, of course, but that could have happened already, quietly and privately. If you notice that your massage partner is feeling well, then you have done a good job of giving a massage. As well, it is important in intuitive crystal massage that you leave time for your partner or client to rest and enjoy the aftereffects. Finally, don't forget the final steps of closing the protective field, purifying the room, and cleansing the massage stones that were used.

A COMPENDIUM OF MINERALS
USED IN MASSAGE

The many different effects that can be produced using stones and crystals of different shapes and sizes is only one factor determining your choice of stone. Equally, if not perhaps more significant, is mineral content—the specific type of mineral being used, which can have a profound effect on the results of a massage.

It is sometimes amazing how different one and the same massage technique feels if we use, for example, orange calcite during one massage, then rose quartz, rock crystal, or sodalite in another session. The differences are enormous, even if the stones are all exactly the same shape. One stone, for instance, might tickle, while another cools, or warms, or vitalizes, or relaxes. The reactions produced are a result of the choice of mineral, and they can vary from person to person.

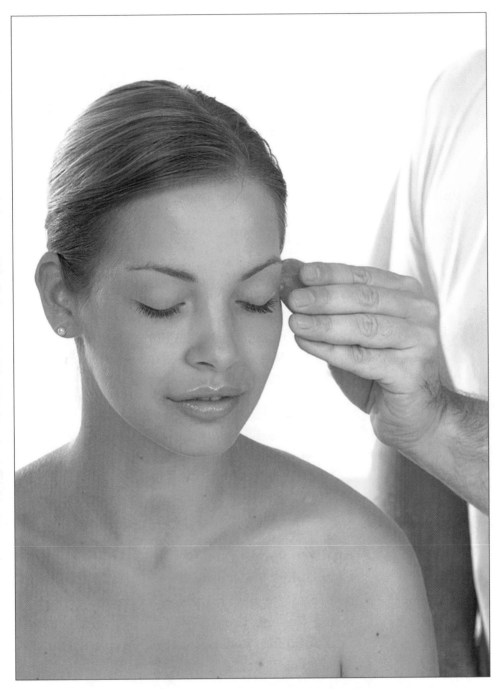

The type of mineral used can have a profound effect on the
results of a massage.

The following list of minerals used in massage and their effects can serve as a useful guide in choosing one mineral over another, depending on the person and the situation. This list does not include all possible qualities and attributes of each mineral, but should give you a sense of some of the general effects observed. All the healing stones and crystals mentioned here are available as massage stones, especially in the aforementioned lens and soap shapes, but also as oloids (intersecting geometric forms, as in many kinds of crystals), disc shapes, and thumb shapes, and as pocket stones and rounded, polished and tumbled stones (worry stones). All of these shapes can be used for intuitive healing stone and crystal massage.

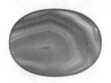

Agate gives a good bodily sensation, a gentle feeling of being enveloped and protected by your own skin. It helps the metabolism of the connective tissue and is therefore good for the skin.

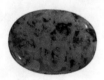

Agate (lace), a more filigree form of agate, is very good for the supply and waste disposal of the connective tissue as well as for the arteries and intestines. It brings finesse, mobility, and spiritual flexibility.

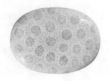

Agatized coral (Petoskey stone) is a rock and a fossil, often pebble shaped, composed of a fossilized rugose coral. It helps to gently reduce deeply rooted tensions. Coral in general helps one cope with difficulties, and with integrating oneself into social groups.

Alabaster (orange) strengthens tissues and loosens stiff muscles. It helps one to define oneself and stabilizes unbalanced psychological states. Orange alabaster also helps heal infections.

Amazonite, a green variety of microcline feldspar, is a wonderful massage stone for joint problems with different causes (stress, rheumatism, infections, liver conditions, etc.). Amazonite also balances moods.

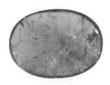

Amethyst eases tension and gives inner peace. More intense massages can churn up the emotions, often bringing out sadness and grief. Physically, amethyst is good for the skin and nerves.

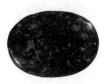

Anthophyllite, which is usually dark hued and can also be green, black, colorless, white, yellow, blue, or brown, is very good for the kidneys and ears. Massages around the ears can help against tinnitus or other ailments. It also helps resolves stress and protect the nerves.

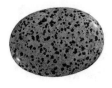

Aplite (Dalmatian stone), intrusive rock in which quartz and feldspar are the dominant minerals, giving it a white, grey, or pinkish cast, has a strengthening, constructive, and emotionally balancing effect—a massage stone for balanced firmness and flexibility, for stable nerves, and for good reaction capabilities.

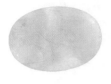

Aquamarine is very good for tired or aching eyes if you massage the area around the eyes with it. Used regularly, it also helps prevent cross-eyedness and regulates near- and farsightedness.

Aventurine, a form of quartz, encourages relaxation and sleep and helps heart conditions, stress, and nervousness. It is also effective for infections, sunburn, and sunstroke if you massage using gentle strokes.

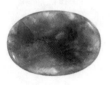

Banded amethyst, a purple variety of quartz whose coloration is due to ferrous iron impurities, relieves tension and headaches, soothes itching and sunburn (rub and pull only lightly for sunburn), and is helpful for people suffering from chronic fatigue.

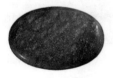

Blue quartz (blue aventurine) cools and calms, helps nervousness, and lowers blood pressure and high pulse rate. It also helps chronic tension and soothes pain.

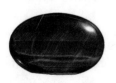

Blue tiger's eye (hawk's eye) brings you "back to earth" in crisis situations and helps you to see things objectively and to attain the proper distance. It eases restlessness, nervousness, shivering, and pain and regulates overactive hormones.

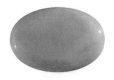

Calcite (blue) both calms and encourages inner stability and security. It is very good for the lymph, skin, colon, connective tissue, bones, and teeth and is especially effective when using to massage the jaw.

Calcite (orange) warms, vitalizes, and brings excellent bodily feelings (coenesthesia; i.e., general awareness of one's own body). It is very effective for the entire abdomen as well as for connective tissue, skin, joints, and bones.

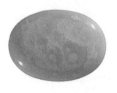

Chalcedony (as blue-banded crystal), a cryptocrystalline form of silica composed of very fine intergrowths of the minerals quartz and moganite, activates body fluids, especially the lymph glands, kidney, and bladder activity; also lowers high blood pressure.

Dumortierite, a fibrous, variably colored aluminum borosilicate mineral, gives serenity and lightness (it's a "take-it-easy" stone). It is helpful for pain, cramps, headaches, nervousness, motion sickness, and even nausea and vomiting.

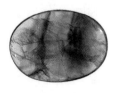

Fluorite (as multicolored rainbow fluorite) is good for the skin, tissues, bones, and joints. It eases chronic tension, enables physical mobility, and helps posture problems. Fluorite activates the nerves.

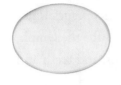

Girasol quartz (girasol opal) is a term some-times mistakenly and improperly used to refer to fire opals, as well as to a type of transparent to semitransparent milky quartz. Used as a massage crystal, it makes you quiet, balanced, open, and able to work under pressure. In massages around the eyes it strengthens vision.

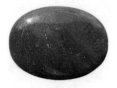

Heliotrope (bloodstone), a form of chalce-dony, is the echinacea of gemstones. It strengthens the body's defenses, eases infections, and helps early heart conditions. Heliotrope helps us define and gather ourselves.

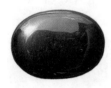

Hematite, the mineral form of iron oxide, gives power and vitality. It vitalizes, making the blood circulate, and warms, making the person active and "burning for action." Physically it encourages hae-matopoiesis (the formation of blood) and oxygen transportation, and provides for vitality here, too.

Jasper (red jasper or brecciated jasper), a form of chalcedony, activates circulation and helps deal with weakness and exhaustion. It circu-lates blood, warms, and gives energy. Red jasper especially boosts courage and the ability to assert oneself.

Jet (lignite), which is not considered a true mineral, but rather a mineraloid, as it has an organic origin (being derived from decaying wood under extreme pressure), is either black or very dark brown and may contain pyrite inclusions. It is very good for mouth, digestion, intestines, skin, joints, and spine. Facial massage with jet can ease bruxism (grinding or clenching of the teeth), while abdominal massage with this stone has a regulating effect on the intestines (helpful for diarrhea).

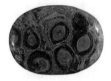

Kambaba jasper (stromatolite), a rare fossilized jasper from Madagascar (commonly called fossilized blue-green algae) is very good for the skin. It opens pores and encourages perspiration and the detoxification that comes with this. It's a very good massage stone to use in the sauna and before purification baths.

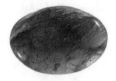

Labradorite, a feldspar mineral, is cooling on the one hand but helps people who are shivering or who are sensitive to the cold. It reduces blood pressure and eases rheumatic conditions.

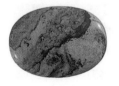

Landscape jasper, an opaque, microcrystalline form of quartz, assists digestion and excretion (stomach, pancreas, and intestines), and strengthens the spleen and the cleansing of connective tissues. Mentally, it gives constancy and endurance.

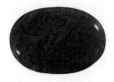

Lapis lazuli is very good for sore throats of any kind, calms the nerves, and has simultaneously both a cooling and a vitalizing effect. It helps us confide in others and to gain control over our lives.

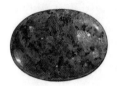

Larvikite (syenite, monzonite, Norwegian pearl granite), notable for its thumbnail-size crystals of feldspar, helps heal heavy emotional disturbances, making you sober and neutral. It also calms the nerves, encourages purification of the tissues, has a cooling effect, and reduces blood pressure.

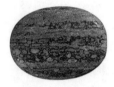

Leopard skin jasper (rhyolite) activates digestion and excretion and helps with skin problems and hardened tissue. It balances activity and rest and improves sleep.

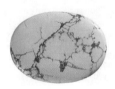

Magnesite has a deeply relaxing effect and helps with cramps and all kinds of pains. It eases headaches, migraines, sore muscles, stomach problems, nausea, back disorders, and shooting pain.

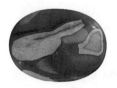

Mookaite, an Aboriginal word meaning "running waters" (it is mined in Australia), gives an overall good body feeling (coenesthesia) because it has simultaneously a relaxing and a vitalizing effect. It makes you soft and strong at the same time, encourages blood purification, and strengthens the spleen, liver, and immune system.

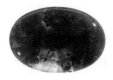

Moss agate (mocha stone), a form of chalcedony that includes minerals of a green color, activates lymph flow and the cleansing of tissue, mucous membranes, and the respiratory tract. It loosens inner tension and is liberating if you feel heavy, depressed, and constricted.

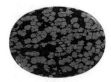

Obsidian (snowflake obsidian) helps pain, mental and physical blocks, and dysfunctions of blood circulation or chronically cold hands and feet. It has a vitalizing and spontaneously motivating effect on the mind.

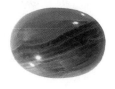

Ocean agate (ocean jasper) contains variably colored orbs (spherical inclusions, or "eyes") that are said to give it protective properties against the "evil eye." It tightens tissue, encourages lymph flow and detoxification, enhances the immune system, eases infections, and retards the growth of cysts and tumors. It gives the courage to face life and have hope.

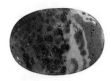

Onyx marble, found in Arizona, preserves fossils dating back to the Neogene period. It is very good for the spine, the intervertebral discs, the meniscus, and joint disorders. It helps in cases of intense mental strain and in situations that develop too quickly.

Petrified wood provides stability and centers. It relaxes and fortifies, strengthens digestion, purifies, and helps in cases of overweight due to a lack of grounding.

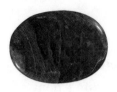

Prase (crysoprase, crysophrase) is a variety of chalcedony that contains small quantities of nickel, giving it a color anywhere from apple green to deep green. It helps with bladder ailments; eases pain, bruises, and swelling; is cooling and reduces fever; and helps with sunburn and sunstroke (stroke gently in such cases). Prase calms hot-tempered types.

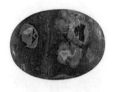

Rainforest jasper (green rhyolite) is very good for the skin and subcutis. It aids purification and therefore eases colds and infections. Mentally, rainforest jasper has a soft, gradual energy and helps us accept ourselves as we are.

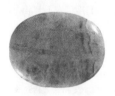

Rhodonite, well known for its beautiful pink and red color, is very good for the muscles, connective tissue, and circulation. It helps heart conditions and aids the healing of scars and old wounds. Rhodonite helps us to let go, to forgive, and to start anew.

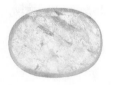

Rock crystal (quartz) cools and refreshes and has a liberating and loosening effect but also revitalizes. It eases pain, opens up the senses, awakens and makes one clear, receptive, and aware.

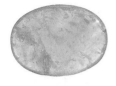

Rose quartz improves senses and overall body feeling. It is good for the heart and aids blood circulation in the tissues. Rose quartz makes you aware of your needs and therefore may be relaxing at one time and stimulating at another. Its energetic hallmark is that of unconditional love that opens the heart chakra.

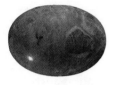

Ruby kyanite, a beautiful combination of ruby and blue kyanite and fuchsite, is very rare but quite valuable in a crystal healing sense. This combination of three minerals helps paralysis, rheumatism, and afflictions of the skin, heart, and back.

Schorl (black tourmaline) is associated with the root chakra and is excellent for grounding and transforming negative energy. It helps to reduce tension and enables a person to be composed and neutral. It alleviates pain and tension in general. In energetic terms, schorl unblocks scar tissue and helps with kinetic disorders, paralysis, and numbness.

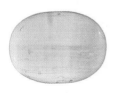

Selenite (fiber gypsum) tightens tissue and eases pain, especially from overexertion. Mentally, it calms you when you are irritable and hyperactive, just when you think you are about to "lose it."

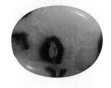

Septarian (dragonstone), a combination of calcite, chalcedony, and aragonite, helps intestinal and skin ailments and hyperacidity. It loosens hardening and tumor growths in tissue and in general helps a person open up. Metaphysically it is excellent for promoting self-caring, caring for others, and caring for Mother Earth.

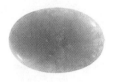

Serpentine (China jade, silver eye) is strongly relaxing and helps nervousness, unease, and the feeling of being unprotected. It alleviates cardiac arrhythmias and kidney, stomach, and menstrual disorders.

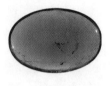

Smoky quartz eases pain and helps reduce tension caused by stress. It is especially effective for headaches, neck and back problems, and tense jaw muscles. Smoky quartz gives strength when someone is under constant pressure.

Sodalite is a stone of logic, rationality, and efficiency. It cools, eases heat sensitivity, reduces fever and blood pressure, and helps sore throats and hoarseness. It liberates you when you have the feeling that you are being prevented from shaping your own life. In crystal healing it is said to be beneficial for the glands, diabetes, digestive system, lymphatic cancer, relieving insomnia, and decreasing calcium deficiency. It is also used in crystal healing for quick relief of head colds.

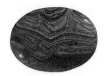

Stromatolite is very good for the intestines and helps the feeling of stomach pressure, also for worries. Stromatolite encourages metabolism and excretion and strengthens connective tissue and skin when used as a massage stone.

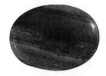

Tiger iron (mugglestone), a combination of hematite, red jasper, and sometimes yellow jasper and golden tiger eye, mobilizes the "tiger in your tank" and gives drive, dynamism, confidence, and a lot of energy and creative power. Tiger iron encourages haematopoiesis and blood circulation and physically activates the circulation. It helps activate exhausted people.

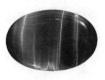

Tiger's eye gives calmness when everything "goes haywire," helps one gather oneself and attain perspective. It eases the consequences of stress and pain and helps one be totally with oneself rather than "beside oneself."

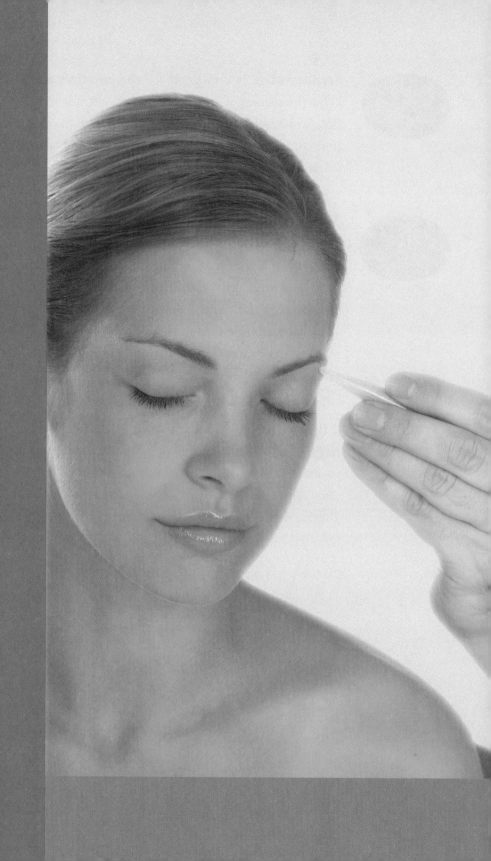

Part 3

Vital Body Massage

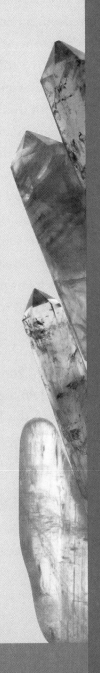

■

In vital body massage we assume that each aspect of our being—every cell, all the tissues and organs, and our entire organism—has consciousness. Our body and every area in it knows exactly what it needs and what does it good. The body has its own intelligence, which is energetic.

WHAT IS THE VITAL BODY?

The term *vital body* refers to the energetic, vibrational body that enlivens and gives essence to the physical body. Vital body massage, therefore, concentrates on the whole person on the energetic level, rather than focusing solely on the physical, mechanical structure, and in this regard it is a true holistic therapy. Vital body massage that uses stones and crystals consists of very gentle touching of the skin with a chosen stone, with the intention of harmonizing and vitalizing the energy field that encircles and penetrates the physical body. This field is also frequently called the *etheric body,* the *vital aura,* the *morphic field,* and the *subtle body*.

This energy field develops from the communication flow between our cells, tissues, and organs, as well as between our physical organism and our soul, mind, and spirit. Every cell in the body, taken on its own, is an autonomous creature with its own consciousness. Each cell controls its own breathing, metabolism, and regeneration. Just imagine if you had to constantly give billions of cells orders; it is far better that they take care of these affairs themselves, isn't it? So insofar as every cell has its own consciousness, it also has a desire to live; it has experiences, knows pain, and knows activity and relaxation. When several cells join together to form tissue, the same consciousness, basically, pertains to this larger entity; the same thing applies when tissues join to form an organ, and again, in the fusion of organs to form an entire organism.

In her presentation on the use of crystal spheres in massage in part 5 of the book, Ursula Dombrowsky provides a valuable description of the body's three systems of communication, and how massage with crystals can play a significant role in improving the flow of intercommunication between these three systems, thus restoring the body to a healthy, harmonious state.

Vital body massage assumes that each aspect of our being—every cell, all the tissues and organs, and our organism as a whole—has consciousness. Our body and every area in it knows exactly what it needs and what it does not need, what does it good and what harms it. The body has its own innate intelligence, which is consciousness, subtle energy.

So given this, why aren't we constantly healthy? Easy: because we listen to our body too rarely! For example, our body signals satiation, yet we keep on eating because it tastes so good (or because we internalized the message not to leave food on our plate). Our body signals fatigue, yet we stay up late, channel surfing. Our body signals thirst, yet instead of serving it hydrating water we serve it soft drinks and coffee, which dehydrate. This list could be extended indefinitely. So it isn't our body's fault when we become ill—it's only doing its best to tell us what it wants. And our usually very forgiving body compensates for many of our "sins" every day; it can do so because it is designed to self-organize.

This organization is only possible through communication: needs have to be expressed, orders have to be transmitted, necessary things must be requested, finished goods must be managed, procedures have to be coordinated, and plans have to be monitored. The logistics of these dimensions can only be accomplished with quick, goal-oriented communication—all the more so because the "organization" (i.e., our body) has trillions of "employees." The physical communication channels, which consist of nerves, blood, and lymph channels, are not sufficient for this load. That's why we also have energetic communication channels, consisting of meridians and biophotons, as well as telepathic networks consisting of synapses.

As well, our energetic communication channels are not limited to our own body. For example, we feel how someone else is doing without anything being said. Our telepathic impulses impart an uneasy feeling when something menacing comes our way, or we feel a sense of joyful well-being when someone is thinking about us in a loving way. A major part of the self-organization of the body is taken care of on this level; that is why thoughts and emotions affect it so directly. And that's not all: the coordination of body, soul, mind, and spirit also takes place this way.

In short, the vital body is the sum of all energetic connections and communication processes in and around our body. The constant exchange via these connections and communications channels is vital to life (Latin: *vita,* "life"). For this reason, this communication and energetic field is called the *vital body;* it is this energetic field that gives us life.

CAN WE PERCEIVE THE VITAL BODY?

Try looking just beyond your skin (for example, over your arm); you will perhaps sense a fine field around your body similar to the reflection of air over a hot road during a summer day, or like the fine white mantle that appears at twilight. This is your vital body, or morphic field, which projects above the physical body by a few centimeters (a little over an inch). You can also feel it when you try running your hand back and forth, gently and empathically, over someone else's skin at a distance of a few centimeters above the surface of the skin. In the same way you can sense fine temperature differences, warm to hot, and cool to even cold, which differ distinctly from the actual skin temperature.

The vital body is similar to a magnetic field. If you approach the skin carefully, a slight resistance that lets your hand spring back can be felt. Ticklish people sometimes react with spontaneous laughter to this kind of touching of the vital body, even without any actual skin contact. You can even make the vital body audible by means of a tuning fork or with resonance spheres; the sound of the resonating tuning fork or sphere changes as you enter and exit the vital body, or when you move it around in it.

Try this exercise to sense your own (or someone else's) vital body, preferably at twilight: Let your eyes blur just beyond your skin; it might help to half-close them. Then run your hands over the body at a distance of a few centimeters (a little over an inch) from the skin, or test the sound changes with a tuning fork or resonance sphere. With a little practice you will be able to sense many nuances.

People who see auras often describe the vital body as a bright, white, or sometimes light yellow field that envelops the body at a distance of two to ten centimeters (about an inch to four inches). Lighter and darker areas can often be seen in this field (it also sometimes seems as if it disappears in the darker areas); the expansion over the borders of the body is not even, either. Light areas reflect energy-rich areas, while dark areas reflect energy-poor areas, which often correspond with the inner state of the respective body zones.

A well-developed ability to see auras lets you see even finer textures in the vital body. You may see countless very fine channels that run from within to without and open in the form of a funnel. These channels are called *nadis,* Sanskrit for "nerve" or "energy channel" in the tradition of ayurveda. They depict the energetic exchange points within the environment. You may also see a gentle flow of inconspicuously flickering and slightly opalizing energy in the whole vital body, comparable to a swirling water surface or the atmospheric swirl in the gas mantle of the planet Jupiter. Countless small swirls or vortices that rotate clockwise and counterclockwise envelop our body. In doing so, they do not remain static; they become smaller and larger, and they change their position and their direction of rotation, too. It is a flexible and lively field that envelops our bodies. The speed of the swirls varies, interestingly enough, and not always in connection with the lighter or darker areas.

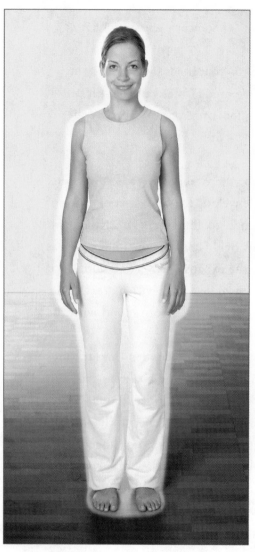

The vital body

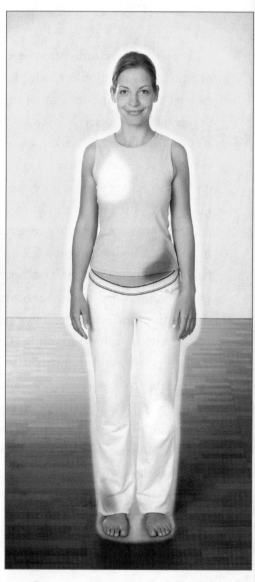

Energy-rich and energy-poor areas
of the vital body

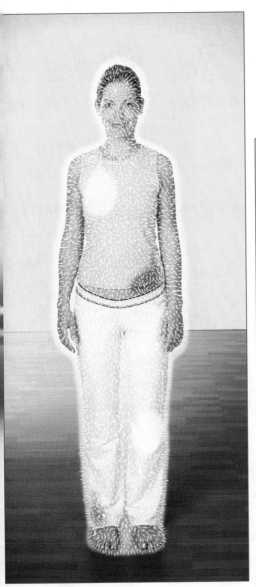

Sheath and nadis

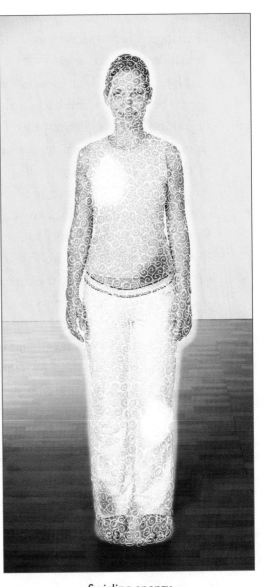

Swirling energy
in the vital body

THE ENERGETIC VORTICES
OF THE BODY

Traditional Chinese medicine says, "Life is change, standstill is death." Accordingly, fast swirls in the vital body signify fast change, slow swirls slow change. Wellness does not depend on our energy levels alone, but rather on *how we maintain our ability to change*. And this willingness to change is not synonymous with either a lot of energy (light areas), or little energy (dark areas).

Nine larger swirls or vortices that are relatively true to their location appear on the front and back of the body, along our central body axis, beginning at the tailbone/pubic bone, all the way up to the parting in our hair at the crown of our head. These swirls are the expression of the nine energy centers called *chakras,* a Sanskrit term that means "turning wheel." They can rotate in different directions, just like the other energy centers. Clockwise movements are, generally, compression and building-up processes; counterclockwise movements are dissolving and decomposition processes. Both are vital. There is no "good" or "bad" associated with the direction of the turn here, whether the rotation is to the right or to the left. Rather, "good" is anything that supports or encourages the natural movement of the vertebrae, while "bad" is anything that retards and blocks energy.

This swirling can also be sensed. Touch the skin very carefully with your index and middle fingers of one hand and start a gentle circling motion. Change direction after two to three circles. You will now notice that the motion is distinctly easier in one direction than the other. Then follow the easier, more effortless direction of rotation. Keep your hand circling while you move it slowly over the skin. Suddenly the rotating direction of your fingers will reverse at some point. Now it becomes easier in the other direction. Soon you will experience another change of direction, and so on as you keep moving your fingers. You see how simple it is to sense the swirls and flows of the vital body? If you continue over your whole body, you will be doing

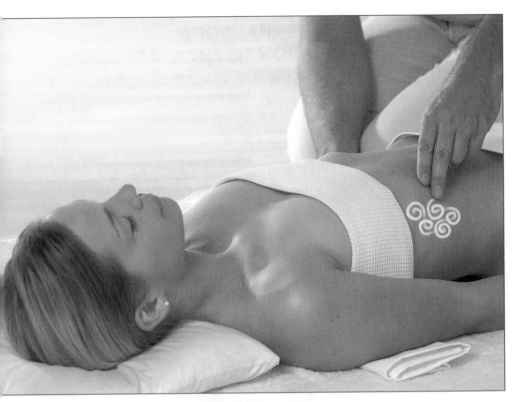

Vital body massage

vital body massage. That's all we have to do. Basically, we're just facilitating the communication within the body.

In vital body massage we follow the natural flow of the vital or morphic field of the body. We do not initiate or force a change, but rather we adjust to the already existing directional flow of energy. We leave the direction up to the body, trusting in its wisdom by supporting it in the way it wants to flow. This improves the communication systems within the body, activating, vitalizing, and strengthening our natural self-healing forces.

THE VITAL BODY
IN RELATION TO THE AURA

The vital body is a part of the *aura,* a word from the Greek meaning "breeze" or "haze." Specifically, it is the inner layer of the aura that expresses the vitality of the body and affects it. Further layers of the

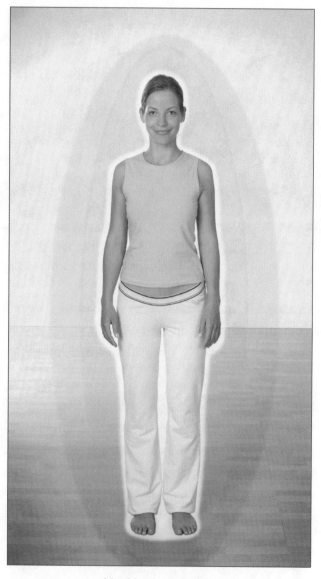

Vital body and aura

aura are the gorgeous emotional body, which can project a good arm's length or more beyond the body and which reflect psychic impulses with its play of colors; and the astral body, which can be room-filling in its clear, clouded, foggy, or free quality, and which reflects our mental state. Finally, there is the invisible causal body, corresponding to our spiritual "space capsule."

Vital body massage does not actively address these additional auric layers. But you can observe that vital body massage influences them indirectly. The glow of the emotional body becomes lighter and more true colored, the mental body becomes clearer and freer, and the person receiving the massage almost always experiences his spiritual space enlarging. In this way, vital body massage reaches not only the physical body but also affects the soul (feelings), the mind (thinking), and the spirit (inner being).

Vital body massage can produce significant metamorphosis in all areas of our being—body, mind, emotions, and spirit—and for this reason it is a holistic massage that simply supports the process of change. These metamorphoses might correspond to that which we really desire in our life. We can see that this is the case by looking at one factor: a dramatic improvement in the person's well-being.

MY BACKGROUND IN VITAL BODY MASSAGE

I have been involved with massage for about half of my life. I first began with a five-year shiatsu massage course in Germany when I was twenty years old, first studying with Martin Stotz and then with Andre Uebele. I then worked as a shiatsu masseur at the end of the 1980s. Around this time I acquired knowledge of vital body massage and other etheric treatment forms from Waltraud Ferrari, a student of the druid Raborne.

The idea of doing vital massage with crystals came to me spontaneously at the beginning of the 1990s, at a time when I had already been using healing crystals for a while in other applications. The crystal wands available to me then, in rock crystal, amethyst, and rose quartz, which I knew of from their application in acupressure massage, made me curious as to what might happen if I were to use them in massaging the vital body. So initially it was simply an experiment among friends—one that had exciting results.

The compendium of crystals and stones found at the conclusion of part 2 of the book provides a valuable overview of the many benefits to be gained by working with the properties of individual stones in vital body massage. Specific stones can be used to address a specific condition or symptom, or rock crystal can be used for general, nonspecific treatments, to relax, vitalize, clear, and liberate. The rock crystal simply gives energy—the correct amount—something we could all use!

The first vital body massages with crystals immediately showed that this is a wonderful way of experiencing the beneficial effects of working with specific gemstones and crystals. In addition to the opening and liberating effects of the massage itself, there is the added sensation that one is filling oneself with the information contained in the stone, as stone type imparts its unique energetic vibrations into the healing process. An added benefit for both the giver and the receiver of the massage is that the physical, psychic, mental, and spiritual qualities of the stone can be sensed directly by both the recipient of the massage and the person offering the massage. In experimenting, we found that many symptoms disappeared almost magically—and in many cases permanently. We were astonished at the powerful effects of this seemingly gentle treatment.

In the early 1990s, as vital body massage was emerging as a via-

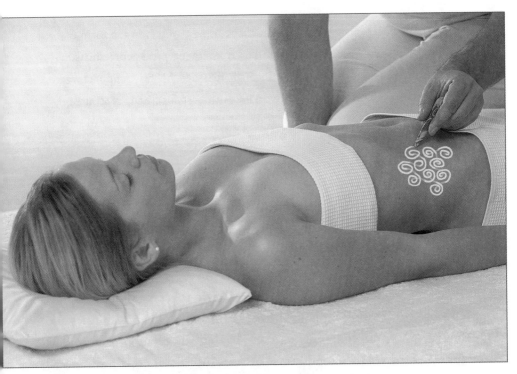

Vital body massage using a crystal stylus

ble therapy, you could really only find quartz crystals in the form of wands or styluses (rock crystal, amethyst, ametrine, smoky quartz, and rose quartz). Ewald Kliegel, a German massage therapist and naturopath who specializes in reflexology, is to be thanked for the fact that by the end of the '90s various additional crystal types were being made into the practical stylus form that he uses for his reflex-zone massages. These new types have been introduced into vital body massage, but the emphasis is still on the use of quartz crystals, especially rock crystal.

Rock crystal massage stylus

Various energetic and massage practices come together in the form of vital body massage: Reiki, which builds energetic protection; shiatsu, which relieves posture issues through massage on the acupuncture points; reflex-zone massage (working with a stylus); and, of course, healing crystal treatments.

I can say from my own experience that after fifteen years of documented use as a practice, vital body massage with healing crystals and gemstones is a viable holistic healing practice that can be administered by anyone if carried out correctly. Of course, as with any form of massage, it is best to receive instruction from an experienced teacher or practitioner.

If you are new to massage in general, or to this type of massage specifically, this chapter explains the basics, including the possibilities and limitations of the vital body massage, so that you can approach it playfully, with partners, friends, or relatives. And if you are a professional massage therapist I believe you will find it quite easy to integrate vital body massage using crystals and stones into your existing repertoire.

A VITAL BODY MASSAGE SEQUENCE

This sequence follows the basic steps found in part 1 of this book; refer back to refresh your memory if necessary.

It is best to administer vital body massage in a warm, quiet room, or outdoors if the temperatures are quite warm and the situation is conducive. Warmth is key, because vital body massage is a massage of the entire body, including its energy sheath. Its effects develop directly on the skin, and sometimes it has a cooling effect because it has a tendency to enlarge the energetic space of the vital body. At the same time know that sometimes the ethereal activation of the vital body has the effect of making the person want to enjoy the freedom and expansiveness that comes with stimulation of the vital body, and so if it is already warm a covering of any kind might be unwanted.

I recommend that this massage be done on the floor, on a firm mattress, or two to three firm, preferably tightly woven wool blankets covered with a sheet. Make sure you have enough room to move around the treatment surface.

> The compendium of stones, located at the end of this part of the book, provides information on which stones are available in stylus, wand, and tumbled forms, the forms that are most suitable to this type of massage.

Crystals and gemstones in the form of wands, styluses, or tumbled stones (longish, rounded, polished "worry" stones), are used in vital body massage. Both the broad, rounded end as well as the pointed, slightly rounded end of the wand and stylus is used; the wide end has a more relaxing, calming effect, and the more pointed end an activating, vitalizing effect. Note that there is no qualitative difference between a wand and a stylus. Choose the shape according to your personal preferences, or else by what is available in the respective crystal type.

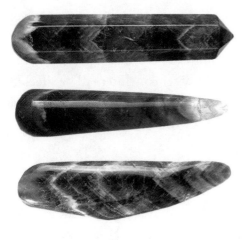

Crystal wand, crystal stylus, and longish tumbled crystal (drop-shaped) of amethyst

We do not use massage oil in vital body massage. This is an important point, as oil changes the skin's surface and diminishes the effects of the stones or crystals. Just let the person you are going to massage find a pleasant position—first in the face-down position and then in the dorsal position—and use pillows, cushions, towel rolls, or other props as needed for comfort. It is best if he is unclad as much as possible because vital body massage only works on the skin. Allow the person a moment of undisturbed peace to settle the body and mind at the beginning.

> Vital body massage only works directly on the skin.

It is important in vital body massage that you protect yourself and the person being treated by surrounding yourselves with light, as described in part 1 of this book, as stones and crystals are powerful energetic transmitters, and foreign, unwanted energy is to be avoided. Tune your intuition by synchronizing your breathing with your counterpart's; this is very helpful because vital body massage is basically steered by the body's intelligence—yours and your counterpart's.

Seat yourself close to the person you are massaging, so that the hand that is holding the stone is turned toward him. If possible it is best if you sit back on your heels, parallel to the body, so that you can look in the direction of the person's head; in this way you can stay upright in a relaxed position and can easily bend forward to carry out the various massage techniques. You will expend the least amount of effort in this position and remain internally collected. As well, you can more readily take a look at the face of the person you are working on in this position so you can get feedback as you proceed.

It is best if you take the wand, stylus, or longish tumbled crystal or stone (which will hereafter be called a *stylus*) in your hand like a pencil, so that you can hold it between your thumb and middle finger and can guide it with your index finger. The back of it will rest in the joint between thumb and index finger, provided it is long enough (which would be ideal). You will need more power to hold and guide

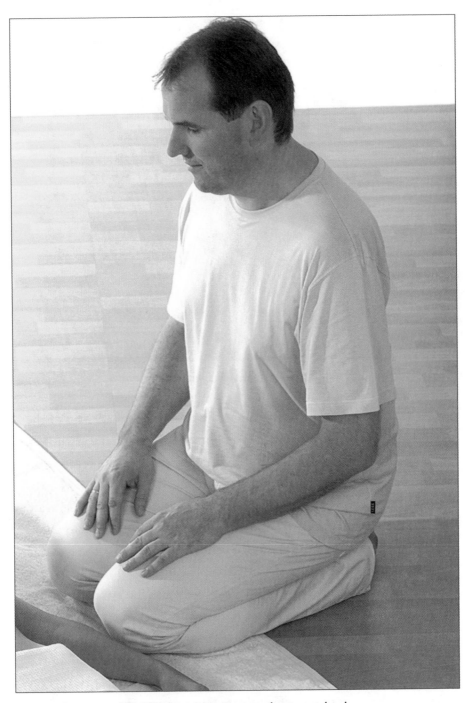

The ideal position is seated on your heels,
parallel to the body

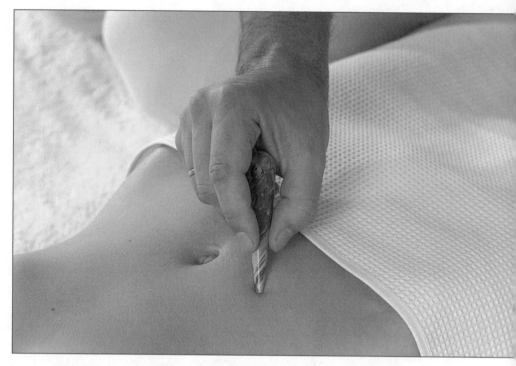

Hold the crystal stylus like a pencil.

it if the stylus is shorter. It is often easier to use the broader tip of the stylus initially if you are new to vital body massage. As already noted, this end has a more relaxing and calming effect, and the reaction to the massage will therefore be more moderate. This is good if you are just learning this practice, because you will still have to concentrate on the technique of the massage and the various sequences. Go ahead and use the more pointed end once you feel more secure; the massage will be livelier then.

Now you are ready to begin the massage. Place the crystal stylus on the skin very, very gently, and let it remain there for a moment. It is a minimal touch, with no pressure whatsoever; on the contrary, lean back a bit internally, just so you have the feeling you are pulling the stylus back if you are in a leaning-forward position. Practice this on your own knee or thigh before the session: sit upright, lean forward, and place the stylus on your skin with a light pressure. Now move it gently, in a circling motion, a couple of times. Now lean back just a few millimeters (this is more an internal than an external feeling), just as if you were ready to lay a pen down at the end of writing a letter. The stylus stays in position naturally in this case, but you pull it back just enough so that you are barely touching the skin, so that there is only a hint of a touch left. Can you feel the difference?

In vital body massage we hover above the entire body, making small circles with the stylus, grazing the skin with just a hint of a touch. More precisely, the circles are actually small, spiraling movements that begin at one point, get larger, and then return to this point in a spiral motion. We wander over the whole body in this circling fashion, always relocating whichever central point we are working from. In doing so we keep changing the direction of the movement, using our intuition to determine whichever direction feels easiest and without resistance.

Though it is possible to give vital body massage without any direct skin contact, by lightly touching in this way, the attention of the person being massaged is directed to the relevant area, which improves the effects and keeps our partner spiritually present. The effects achieved through this light touch are more physical, meaning that it is more a stimulation of the reflex zones. Harder contact with the stylus feels good, too, but it is a different kind of massage technique form than is covered in this book.

> It is very important in massaging the vital body that contact with the stylus is really minimal—very gentle, just a hint of pressure. The gentler, the better. Let your intuition be your guide.

As long as you are in tune with your client, you can rely on your intuition to guide your hand in terms of which direction to proceed. Always gradually massage the whole body, or the entire area if you are focusing on just a part of the body. You can either proceed intuitively in this fashion or you can follow a sequence. The conventional

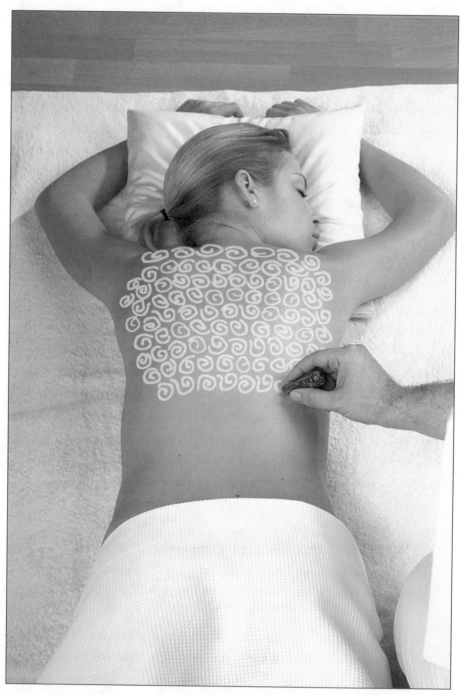

Motion of the crystal stylus
in small spiraling movements

sequence (rarely carried out in intuitive massage work) would be to begin with the client lying in the prone, face-down position; then starting at the crown of the head, run down the neck, shoulders, back, buttocks, and legs (one after the other), to the soles of the feet and the tips of the toes, using circling movements of the stone or crystal. Then, with the client supine and face up, you change your position and massage upward, starting at the tips of toes, then the feet, legs, pelvis/abdomen, and chest, along the arms to the fingertips (one arm then the other). The arms are stretched out to the side with palms upward as you massage from armpit to fingertips. The arms are then positioned loosely next to the body, palms down, as you massage back to the shoulders.

Then change your position and sit above the head of the person you are massaging. You can now proceed to massage from one shoulder, along the neck and behind the ears, up to the top of the skull (first one shoulder, then the other). From there move over the forehead to the temples and ears, then from the base of the nose over the closed eyelids to the zygomatic bone and hinge of the jaw, and finally from the nose, over the cheeks, around the mouth, and over the chin. These pathways in the face are only clues, though. This sequence can be modified according to what your intuition and experience tell you. As a conclusion, lay the stylus on the person's third eye, the chakra point between the eyebrows, for twenty to thirty seconds. Listen to your intuition here as you should do throughout the massage; a good conclusion brings grace to the whole process.

Always allow yourself to be led by the vital body when you apply the circling, spiraling movements of the stylus. The best way to achieve this is through the attitude that it is not you making the movements, but rather you are just letting them happen, as if dictated by the person's energetic body. If you have doubts, try switching hands or changing to the other side to see if it is easier to circle to the right or to the left. The easier movement, which will reveal itself, is always the correct one. You will achieve a free flow after a while

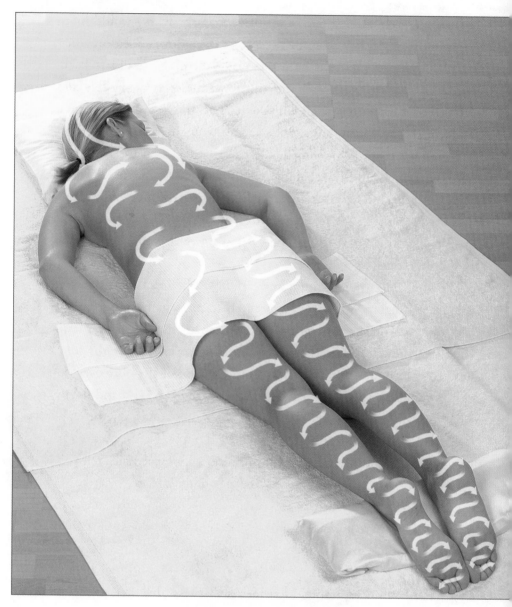

The sequence of vital body
massage often begins with the
client lying face down

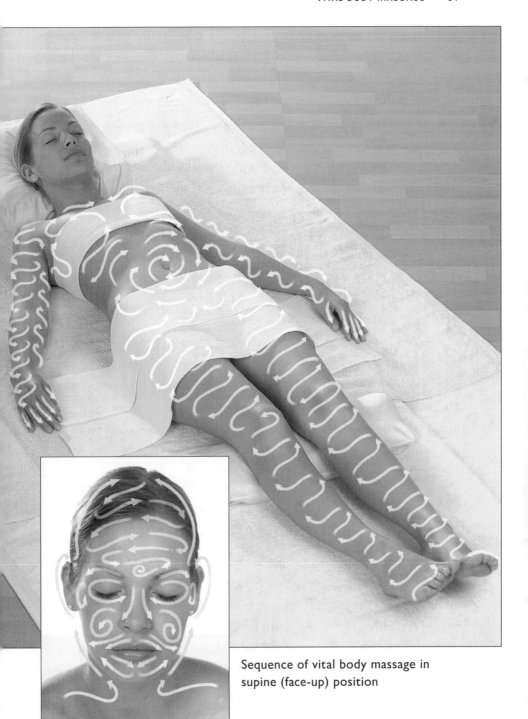

Sequence of vital body massage in
supine (face-up) position

and the movement will seem to take place by itself. Your hand simply circles clockwise one time, counterclockwise the next, clockwise, counterclockwise, and so forth, as you move the stone over the body. You can basically just observe, keeping an eye on the whole process. Stay in contact, too, with the person you are massaging by simply observing his reaction. Be sure to give any emotional releases space to be expressed. The vital body massage ends either after the completion of the massage of the whole body or at the moment of uplift, as described in part 1 of this book.

It is best to stay present, spiritually and physically, after the completion of the vital body massage. Remain quiet and be aware of how the person you just worked on is doing. As it is an energetic massage it is very important that you "trade back" any energy that might have been exchanged between you and the person, and that you free any lingering energy that might have gotten caught in the room. This can be done mentally as long as you sit quietly waiting next to the person whom you massaged. There is enough time afterward for an exchange or feedback, if the person so desires to initiate such a dialogue. Finally, it is essential that you cleanse the crystal stylus used following the session.

BENEFITS OF
VITAL BODY MASSAGE WITH STONES

The improved communication between body, mind, intellect, and spirit that results from vital body massage opens us to understanding more clearly what is good for our bodies. That is why it is important to observe which needs and wishes arise in the period after a vital body massage—and to follow them! If we suddenly have an urgent wish to sleep, then we probably need it. (So, off to bed!) We sometimes do not even notice at first that our sleep disturbances have disappeared. It is worth following an urge if we suddenly feel one—to do more sports, to eat certain foods, to engage in certain hobbies, to have contact with

Vital Body Massage
Sequence Points to Remember

1. Find a comfortable position for the person being treated and enough warmth.
2. Arrange the crystals and stones that will be used for the session.
3. Center yourself, establish a protective boundary, and generate intuition and empathy.
4. Take an upright posture (e.g., sitting on your heels, leaning forward slightly to treat).
5. Hold the crystal stylus in your hand like a pencil.
6. Lay the crystal on the skin very gently, and circle delicately on impulse. Massage the entire body, alternating the circling directions.
7. Let alternating spiraling movements happen; see which direction is easier.
8. Possible sequence of the massage: back of the head, back, buttocks, back of the legs, feet, front of the legs, pelvis, abdomen, chest, arms, head, face.
9. Stay in contact and look for feedback; ask the person how he is doing if necessary.
10. End the vital body massage at the completion of the massage of the whole body or at the moment of uplift.
11. Following the massage, stay present, observe, and ask about any needs.
12. Trade back possible taken-over energy, dissolve the protective sheath, and cleanse any energy still stuck in the room.
13. Take time for feedback and conversation if the person so desires.
14. Deliberately drop the therapist role after the person leaves.
15. Cleanse the crystal stylus, and clean the room, if necessary.

certain people, or to talk things out or settle something that has been nagging at us. We are often led to what will help us or heal us following a vital body massage.

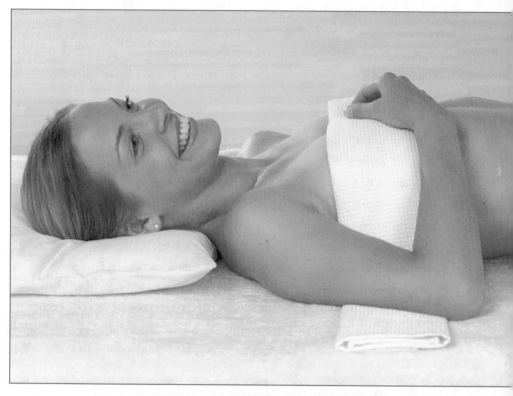

Vital body massage opens us to understanding
more clearly what is good for our bodies.

Vital body massage with healing crystals increases the energy flow in
the vital body and thus improves communication between the body,
soul, intellect and spirit. In most cases this is noticeable at first in
terms of an improved coenesthesia. Vital body massage doesn't solve
all the problems a person may have straight away; it does not "work
wonders" (even though it feels wonderful), but it can facilitate more
long-term healing.

The goal of this kind of energetic body massage is the harmonizing of the vital body. This is attained in the short term through
the massage, but its effects stabilize only if we accordingly shape our

life harmoniously. The return to an inharmonious state shows us all those particular areas that are sources of disharmony; or maybe we have insights into what could prolong and stabilize this harmonious state. If we get vital body massage on a regular basis, it can contribute to beneficial change and a reorganization of one's life—as long as we follow through on the respective impulses and implement them. The ability to implement them, too, is improved by vital body massage. The swirling and circling of the vital energy indicates change, mutability, and willingness to change. We strengthen our capacity to make changes in our life by supporting this turning and swirling energy. That is why vital body massages make you more flexible, both physically and spiritually.

> A good image for the effect of vital body massage is water: it is versatile and mobile, and can adapt to any form—and it still keeps its balance anytime, anywhere, effortlessly!

Physically, improved vitality appears as more stable health. But this does not usually manifest immediately. The things that have to be changed to achieve this kind of harmony show up first; for this reason, certain disorders appear or become more readily discernible in the beginning. But then, layer by layer, successive blockages and disorders dissolve as the process continues. This process, of course, is facilitated by regular vital body massage.

By adding gemstones and healing crystals (in the form of wands, styluses, or longish tumbled stones) to a vital body massage, we give the massage an added dimension and direction. The results are determined by the nature and properties of the stones or crystals used, so we should therefore think carefully about which ones we choose. And if there is any doubt, if you do not know or are just unsure which crystal fits best, a good choice is always the neutral rock crystal.

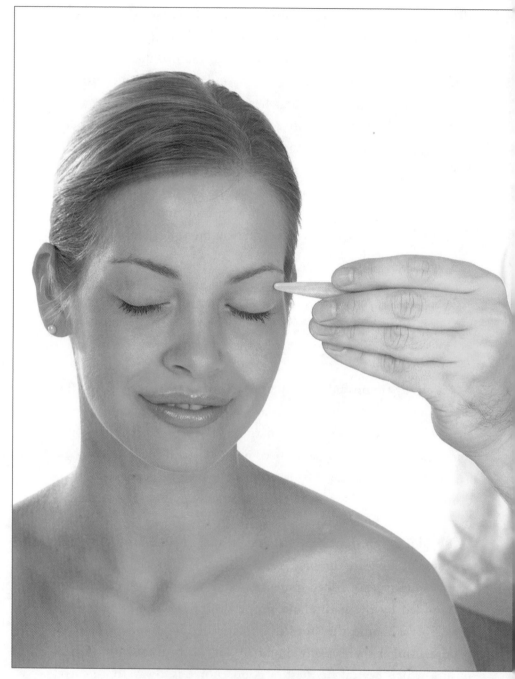

Gemstones and crystals give a massage
an added dimension and direction.

Vital body massage that incorporates healing crystals has an effect that can be perceived immediately in terms of a sense of well-being and spiritual freedom and improved coenesthesia, and a medium- to long-term effect in terms of increasing one's flexibility toward change, more stable health, an upsurge of new impulses, and new dynamics and order in life. The long-term aspects become even stronger if we get vital body massage on a regular basis.

INDICATIONS AND CONTRAINDICATIONS FOR VITAL BODY MASSAGE

■ **Massage when you are well.** What basically applies for all types of crystal and stone massage—and for massage in general—applies here: do not give a vital body massage if you are not well yourself or if you are not in a good mood. It is not only your hands that have an effect, especially in any kind of massage that deals with the energetic body, but also your moods and thoughts. Crystals and gemstones are extremely sensitive to mood. A massage given when you are tired, reluctant, or sick can weaken both the person treating and the person being treated. Massage only if you are feeling well and if you feel like doing it. You can obtain wonderful results with vital body massage with healing crystals as long as you observe the rules.

■ **Follow the body's own innate energy.** The speed and duration of a massage is up to you, but one rule is unchanging: never go against the natural direction of the flow of the energy swirls or vortices in the vital body. Always follow the easier direction, or the direction in which energy appears to flow on its own. Bear in mind that, as we have already said, there is no "good" or "bad" regarding movements to the right or the left. And remember also to follow the energy swirls lightly and gently. You do not need to push; in fact, move your crystal stylus like a blade of grass over water.

■ **Use your intuition in choosing which crystal or stone.** You can always rely on the help of a pendulum or a divining rod, or you can muscle test for the right stone. And when in doubt, choose a rock crystal.

■ **Pregnancy.** Not all stone types are appropriate during pregnancy. Experience shows that agate (pregnancy protection), amethyst (peace, relaxation), onyx marble (against back disorders), rock crystal (universal), calcite (bones, growth, development), chalcedony (for lymph congestion or edema), heliotrope (differentiation, protection against infections), rose quartz (feelings of empathy), and serpentine (relaxation) are all good stones to use. Be especially careful in the last two months of pregnancy, especially if the pregnancy has not progressed smoothly. Vital body massage is recommended directly before birth, though, because it can facilitate childbirth; magnesite or serpentine can help to relax the pelvic floor at this time.

■ **Chronic illness.** Caution is necessary in cases of acute or chronic illness. Vital body massage should only be administered by experienced doctors or practitioners in this case. This applies, for instance, even to colds when there is a high fever.

A COMPENDIUM OF MINERALS RECOMMENDED FOR USE IN VITAL BODY MASSAGE

The following crystal types are found as wands, styluses, or longish tumbled stones—the best forms to use in vital body massage. This does not mean that these are the only healing crystals that can be used in vital body massage, simply that this group of minerals would form a good basic collection to choose from for those wanting to try out this type of massage.

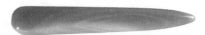

Agate is generally available as a crystal stylus, not as a wand. It is applied in vital body massage mainly for protection, security, good sleep, and groundedness. Vital body massages with agate imparts inner security and stability. Physically, it assists digestion, excretion, and connective tissue and skin repair.

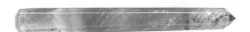

Amethyst is mainly available as a crystal wand. **Banded Amethyst (chevron amethyst),** which is also well suited for vital body massage, is obtainable in stylus form and in the form of longish tumbled stones, or "drops." Amethyst gives inner peace and helps overcome mourning and grief. It relaxes, but makes you alert and aware at the same time. Physically, vital body massage with amethyst eases strong tension and headaches.

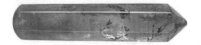

Ametrine (trystine, bolivianite), a mixture of amethyst and citrine with zones of purple and yellow or orange, was available as a crystal wand in the past but is harder to find these days. Its qualities are similar to amethyst, but it makes you happier and more dynamic. Physically, vital body massage with ametrine is very good for the nerves.

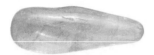

Aquamarine is unknown as a crystal wand or stylus and found only very rarely as a longish tumbled stone. A lens-shaped stone could be substituted. Aquamarine gives lightness and serenity, accompanied by discipline and endurance. It imparts the feeling that things can be accomplished "in the blink of an eye." Physically, aquamarine regulates growth and hormonal balance and helps allergies, especially hay fever. Vital body massage with aquamarine also has a positive effect on the eyes, especially for cross-eyedness and near- and farsightedness.

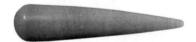

Aventurine is available as a crystal wand and as a stylus. Vital body massages with aventurine are excellent for problems with falling asleep. Aventurine helps to turn off the thoughts circling in your mind, as well as to diminish stress and nervousness. Physically, aventurine is very good for the influence of radiation, including solar radiation.

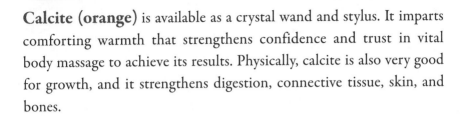

Calcite (orange) is available as a crystal wand and stylus. It imparts comforting warmth that strengthens confidence and trust in vital body massage to achieve its results. Physically, calcite is also very good for growth, and it strengthens digestion, connective tissue, skin, and bones.

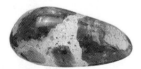

Chalcedony (as blue-banded crystal) used to be available as a crystal stylus. It is rarely available as of this writing because of a scarcity of the raw material. The original stone, before cutting, has to be much larger than the stylus. Longish tumbled stones may be used as an alternative. Chalcedony makes things flow when we feel inhibited and limited. It makes us open, communicative, and alert. Physically, vital body massage with chalcedony boosts the flow of body liquids, especially lymph. The activity of the glands, kidneys, and bladder is also often stimulated.

Fire opal is not available as a crystal wand or stylus. There are, very rarely, longish tumbled stones of fire opal in bedrock that are ideally suited for vital body massage, however. Fire opal bestows wonderful erotic massages. It vitalizes; makes one open-minded, cheerful, and fond of life; and makes sexuality fun. Physically, it gives power and the ability to perform and boosts potency and fertility.

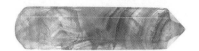

Fluorite (as multicolored rainbow fluorite from China) is a classic crystal wand and stylus. It is unfortunately very fragile and therefore must be treated carefully. Fluorite gives (depending on the situation) structure and order to life or makes one more flexible, freer, and more open. Vital body massage with fluorite also helps stress and learning and concentration disorders. Physically, it improves posture and mobility and helps coughing, hoarseness, and irritated or diseased mucous membranes.

Heliotrope is available as a crystal wand. Vital body massage with heliotrope strengthens the ability to define oneself and to "get a grip" on life. Physically it stimulates the immune system, which is the reason vital body massage with this crystal is very good for colds and the beginning of illnesses. It also has an easing effect in heart conditions.

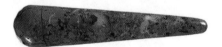

Jasper (red jasper, brecciated jasper) can be found in both wand and stylus shapes. Vital body massage with red jasper makes one very active and dynamic. Jasper gives power and drive, but one should be discerning because sometimes it can make a person agitated and impatient. Physically, it stimulates circulation and helps constant weakness and fatigue.

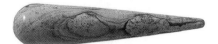

Landscape jasper is mainly available in the form of crystal styluses, rarely as wands. Yellow-brown landscape jasper gives quiet reliability and endurance (in contrast to red jasper). Physically, landscape jasper assists digestion and excretion as well as the cleansing of connective tissues, so it therefore eases allergies.

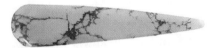

Magnesite is available in both wand and stylus shapes. It has a relaxing effect and helps cramps and various pains. Vital body massages with magnesite make one patient and calms agitation and fearfulness. Physically, it helps headaches, migraines, sore muscles, stomach disorders, nausea, backache, and joint pains.

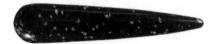

Obsidian (snowflake obsidian) is available in both wand and stylus shapes. It helps pain and mental and physical blockages as well as the consequences of accidents and injuries. It also stimulates circulation and gives internal warmth if there is a tendency toward chilliness and cold feet and hands.

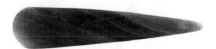

Onyx marble has recently come onto the market in the form of wands and styluses. Onyx marble's inner effects are that of releasing in situations of constant challenge, and it is simultaneously calming and constructive in vital body massage. Physically, it is very good for spinal problems, intervertebral discs, meniscus, and joint conditions.

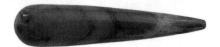

Prase is sometimes available as a crystal stylus. It works very well for swelling, bruises, and other pain; eases solar radiation effects, including sunburn and sunstroke; and helps heat sensitivity as well as the consequences of overheating.

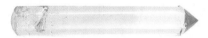

Rock crystal is the classic crystal wand and stylus and a good all-around choice in vital body massage. Longish tumbled stones are not rare either. It can be used practically universally as a neutral, clear quartz and can be unreservedly recommended for first experiments with vital body massage. Rock crystal simply gives the right amount of energy and stimulates clarity. Vital body massages with rock crystal are very liberating.

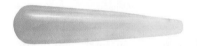

Rose quartz is also one of the classic crystal wands and styluses. It makes one sensitive and empathic and encourages cheerfulness, helpfulness, and empathy. Vital body massage with rose quartz helps many heart ailments (especially cardiac arrhythmia) and sexual problems (caused by tension and pressure to perform), and boosts fertility.

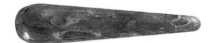

Ruby kyanite, a beautiful combination of ruby and blue kyanite and fuchsite, is rare as a crystal stylus. If you can find one, this stone, composed of the three aforementioned minerals, eases tension due to stress and extreme pressure. It eases pain, encourages good sleep, and gives serenity and the feeling of protection. Physically, it is very good for paralysis, rheumatism, infections, skin diseases, and heart and back disorders.

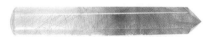

Rutilated quartz is available as a crystal wand. Vital body massage with it loosens tightness and eases tension and anxiety, and it enhances the sense of a wide, free space. It also lightens moods, dissolves fears, and gives a feeling of security and strength. Physically, rutilated quartz encourages cell regeneration and helps with many stubborn illnesses, especially bronchitis and illnesses of the respiratory tract.

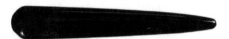

Schorl (black tourmaline) is available in both stylus and wand shapes. Naturally grown slim crystals are sometimes round-polished at the base to make wands. Schorl allows one to reduce internal tension and to become energetically more permeable. Because of this, it also helps to protect against the influence of electrosmog and also against energetic and mental attacks. Massage with it balances energetic differences in the vital body, strengthening it, and it gives a feeling of protection. Schorl helps us be neutral in conflicts and makes us even-tempered. It eases pain and tension and helps unblock energy around scar tissue; it also helps numbness.

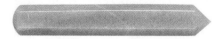

Serpentine (often under the commercial name China jade) is available as both a crystal wand and a stylus. It helps with nervousness, restlessness, fluctuations of mood, and the feeling of not being protected. Vital body massage with serpentine is very relaxing, and it can therefore help when it is difficult to reach orgasm as a result of tension. Physically, massage with this crystal helps cardiac arrhythmia and kidney, stomach, and menstruation disorders.

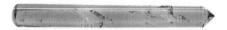

Smoky quartz is a classic crystal wand choice, like the other crystal quartzes. It has been used as an anti-stress stone for a long time in vital body massage. Smoky quartz quickly helps relieve tension caused by stress and pain but at the same time also strengthens one's own ability to work under pressure so that one does not become stressed so easily. It also helps with solar radiation effects and strengthens the nerves.

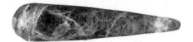

Sodalite is available as both a crystal wand and a stylus. Vital body massage with it is cooling; therefore, it eases heat sensitivity, reduces fever and blood pressure, and helps sore throats and hoarseness. Sodalite helps one attain the space and freedom to experience what one would like to. It supports you in being true to yourself, to change behavior patterns, and to work consistently on your own development.

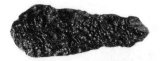

Tektite is available neither as a crystal wand nor a stylus, but in its natural form it is a somewhat furrowed drop, so it is suitable, as such, for vital body massage. Tektite frees and helps to let go; it gives a strong feeling of freedom and detachment at the same time. Tektite can, therefore, be used particularly when we feel that we are ensnared by many things and life is too tight and suffocating. Tektite also helps to compensate for the effects of electrosmog and accelerates healing processes.

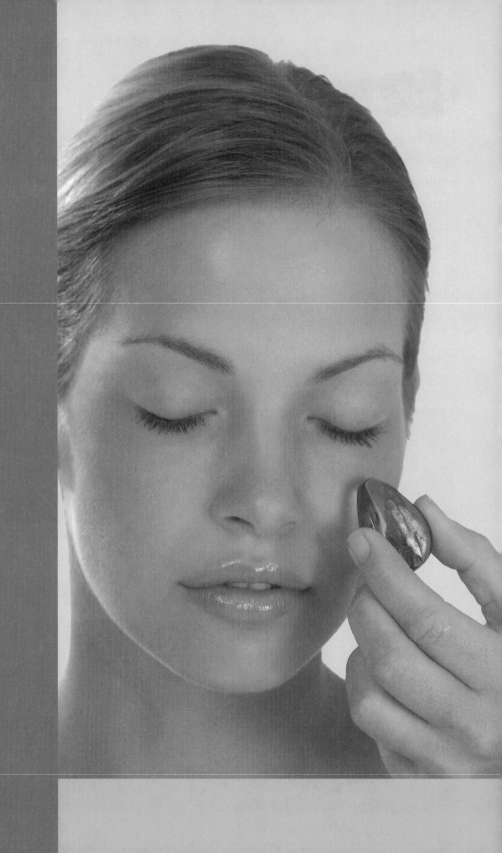

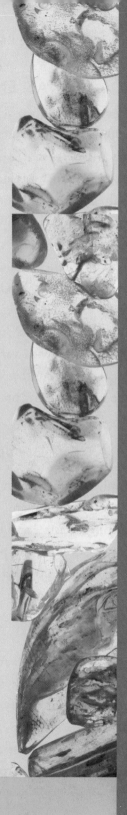

Part 4
Harmonizing Massage with Amber

■

By Hildegard Weiss

Amber is unique. As petrified resin, it has distinctly different properties compared to crystals and gemstones, which are composed of minerals. That is why massage with amber is a particularly effective healing massage in its own class.

AN ENCOUNTER WITH AMBER

The use of amber in harmonizing massage came to my attention in 2002 at a crystal healing symposium in Idar-Oberstein, Germany, when I witnessed a demonstration of its use by Thorsten Vorbrodt. At this point I was already familiar with healing crystal massages, and I already knew about vital, or morphic field, massage, among other practices, through my training with Michael Gienger. As well, I had experience in the use of crystals in massage treatments with my clients for their various ailments, and the wonderful results confirmed everything that Michael had been teaching. So the possibilities of using a special amber stone in massage work swiftly caught my attention, as amber has special electromagnetic vibrations that lend it to healing on a wide variety of levels. Subsequently, in using amber and, in so doing, confirming its properties, something new evolved out of the sum of all my previous experiences.

PROPERTIES OF AMBER

Amber is noted in metaphysics to give a soothing, light energy that is both calming and energizing at the same time. It is said to help manifest desires and heighten intellectual abilities, clarity of thought, and wisdom. It is reputed to cleanse its environment by drawing out negativity, and to relieve physical pain the same way. It is used mystically to bring the energies of patience, protection, psychic shielding, romantic love, sensuality, purification, balance, healing, and calmness. Amber is excellent in crystal healing for inner child work and past life work. Amber is associated with the solar plexus chakra and sometimes the sacral chakra. Mystical lore says that amber is beneficial for purifying the body, headaches, bone problems, heart problems, circulation, ears, hearing problems, endocrine system, fibromyalgia, intestinal/digestive disorders, kidney, bladder, lungs, and general healing purposes. Note that healing crystal meanings are spiritual supports to healing and are not prescriptions or health care information.

A HARMONIZING MASSAGE SEQUENCE WITH AMBER

I always use a wide, comfortable massage table for treatments. My clients feel very good on it, and my body can remain relaxed while I massage in both sitting and standing positions. You can massage on the floor, of course, if you do not own such a table. I always make sure that the temperature in the room is comfortable for the client; I keep a blanket handy and play quiet, relaxing background music. In addition, I relax the client's knees with a knee-roll if desired, and begin the massage by placing small pieces of amber in both hands for the person to hold.

The massage begins at the feet, with the client lying on his or her back; I remain seated during this portion of the massage. The massage can be administered with or without massage oil (jojoba, St. John's wort, etc.). I find that with amber, the massage is often experienced as being even more enjoyable with oil—there's something about the contact between the resinlike stone and a good-quality natural oil that facilitates the energy of the amber. I take both heels in my hands and become aware of the body's rhythm through the client's breathing or through the pulse at the ankles. I then attune myself to this rhythm and relax the feet with various loosening-up exercises, if necessary (for example, rubbing the upper side toward the toes, circling the ankles with the fingertips, light pulling of the individual toes, both feet at the same time). The feet are subsequently placed back on the bed in as relaxed a state as possible, so that I can reach the bottom and inside of the foot comfortably. I massage the soles of the feet over the chakra zones there with gentle circling motions of the amber. I find that with amber as well as with other stones, the easier direction of rotation is always the right direction. Trust your instincts as you move the stones to find the way in which it feels smoothest, without effort.

Through this healing massage with amber, use a light touch, circling any given area, as described in Michael Gienger's "Vital Body Massage" sequence found in part 3 of this book.

The chakra zones on the soles of the feet in stone massage correspond approximately to the zones delineated in reflexology massage. You can harmonize the individual organs by massaging these points.

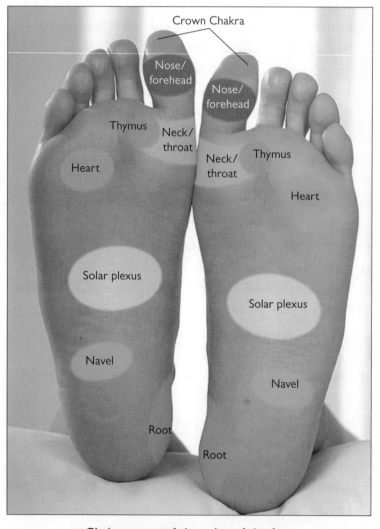

Chakra zones of the soles of the feet

Your client's abdominal noises will confirm the relaxation of the individual organs. This is how you will know that contact with the person has been established, and the person will subsequently visibly relax.

I massage both soles of the feet simultaneously, slowly and equally, with the amber. Retain the massage direction as shown in the picture. The duration of the massage of the respective points is up to the person massaging. You can trust your feelings to guide you, while observing your client's reactions.

You will follow this by proceeding to the top of the foot, from the toes to the ankle; once again, work both feet simultaneously. Pay special attention to the ankles, inside and outside; they should be gently encircled by the amber.

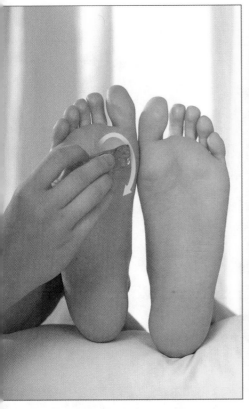

Amber massage of the soles of the feet

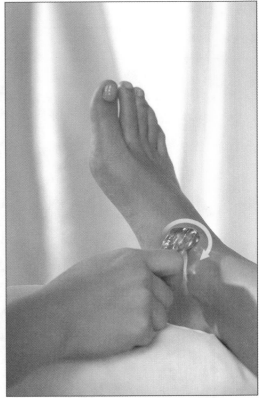

Amber massage of the ankle

Now each of the legs is massaged individually. Leave the one piece of amber lying on the ankle of the resting leg as you turn your attention to the opposite leg; you might need to help it stay there by draping a towel over the foot. The opposite leg is now massaged, starting at the ankle and working up to the knee. I always try to stay in physical contact with my client using both of my hands. Before I start working on the second leg, I place the amber on the knee of the leg I have just finished. It stays there until the second leg has been massaged up to the knee with the amber that was resting on the ankle. After that I place the amber on this knee, too, before proceeding to the knees. The knees are massaged simultaneously, once again with circling movements. Toxins that can sometimes lead to arthritis tend to accumulate in the knee area; attention to the knees activates the circulation and dissolves possible waste products.

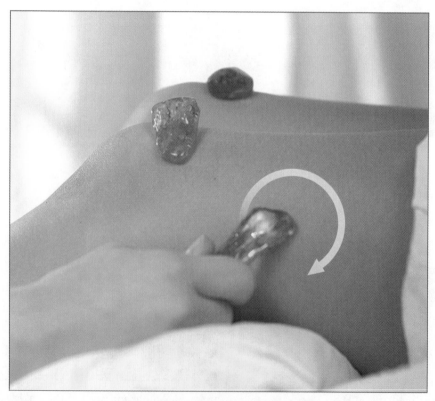

Amber massage of the thigh

Now on to the thighs. They are massaged in the same way as the lower legs, one at a time. The amber pieces should be left resting in the middle of the thigh at the end of the massage of each leg. If they haven't been up to this point, the legs should now be covered to hold the activated warmth.

Next, the hands and arms are massaged individually with amber in the same fashion as the legs and feet: first, the palms of the hand from the carpus joint (wrist) to the tips of the fingers; then the back of the hand to the carpus joint. The amber rests on the carpus joint of one hand until the massage of the other hand is complete. Leave the amber on the wrist of the resting arm and continue up the forearm of the first arm.

The next point of rest is the elbow joint. In general, we do not pay nearly enough attention to the elbow. Just imagine if you had to work at the computer or drive a car without your elbow joints . . .

There are two advantages to setting a point of rest here at the elbow: (1) we direct our attention to this important joint ("energy follows attention," in shamanic wisdom); and (2) we activate blood and oxygen distribution in this joint area with our light, circling, purposeful motions with the amber. Here again, leave a piece of amber on the first elbow joint while massaging the second one. Then place the piece of amber on the second elbow and continue by switching back to the first arm and working up to the shoulder.

The next point of rest is the shoulder joint. Our shoulder joints are important because, among other things, they establish the nerve connection between the head/body and the arms. As well, the shoulders are used in writing, eating, turning the head, carrying something, sleeping, and so forth. It is not for nothing that we use the expression "to shoulder something"! So pay particular attention to the shoulder joints, using light, circling, purposeful motions on each shoulder with the amber. When you've completed one shoulder joint, leave the amber resting there while working on the second shoulder joint.

So at this point we have activated the energy in the limbs and guided it through the body, up to the shoulders. We have also given

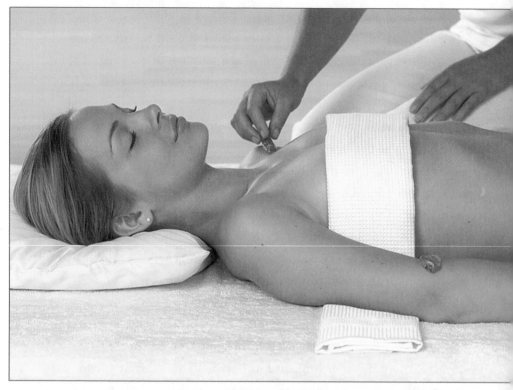

Amber massage of the arms

the inner organs attention with the chakra massage of the soles of the feet. We now turn to the easily overlooked chest muscles and their ligaments. Massage the area above the chest, to the shoulder joints, with the amber in both hands.

Then follow this by massaging the neck muscles on both sides of the neck, out to the shoulder joints. Do *not* massage the front of the neck because of the sensitivity of the larynx and thyroid gland.

At this point I now glide the flat of my hands, palms up, under the supine upper part of the body of my person as far as I can downward. I then make fists and run them up to the shoulders along both sides of the spine. This action is very relaxing for a tense back. I repeat this a few times.

I now lay the amber onto the cheekbones and take my client's head into my hands at the sides very gently, resting here awhile. Both my

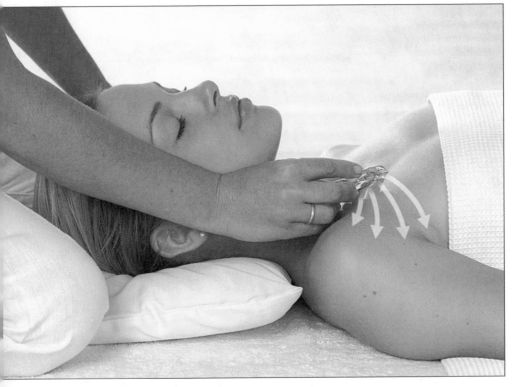

Massaging across the chest

own and the client's attention is now directed to the head region. While this is going on, the rest of the body can be covered, if desired. I then quietly and slowly take my hands away, leaving time for the person to notice the difference in the position of the head. She can now enjoy the facial massage in a much more relaxed state.

I begin to massage the amber over the cheekbones toward the ears with small, circling motions.

I lay a stone on the chin after this. I massage from the tip of the nose to the hairline with another stone. The motion ends in the air; in this way I prevent possible energy concentration in the head. Note that the massage motions on the head are repeated several times, depending on the situation.

Then I proceed with both stones, beginning under the lips. I massage the lower jaw to the jaw joint, on both sides of the face, with

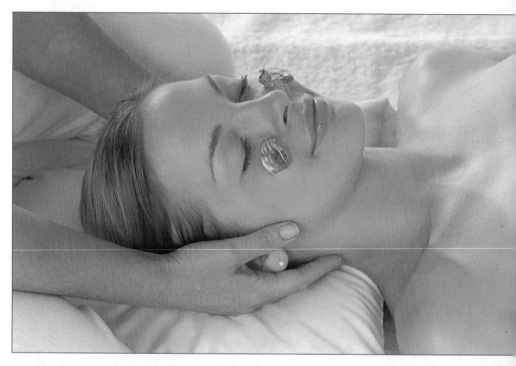

Letting the head rest in the hands

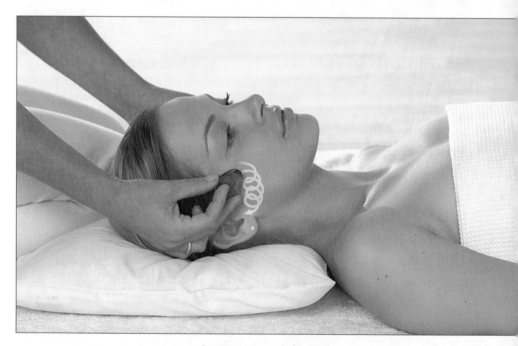

Circling toward the ear

gentle motions. I then begin on the upper jaw above the lips, and massage to the side, toward the jaw joint.

The amber is then reapplied at the outer point of the eyebrows. Massage around the eyes to the root of the nose, in small circles, and from there along both sides of the nose downward, over the corners of the mouth to the chin, then slowly back to the jawbone.

The next point of application is the root of the nose. I massage the forehead toward the hairline, synchronously.

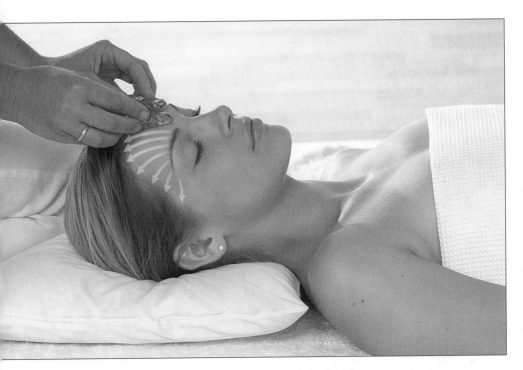

Synchronous rubbing toward the hairline

I then lay the stones to one side and conclude the massage by gently pulling both earlobes at the same time.

Body contact is kept for a while by cupping my opened hands under the person's head at the neck. The person's deep inhaling and exhaling signals the point of uplift, where the massage ends.

Now I let the client rest for at least eight minutes.

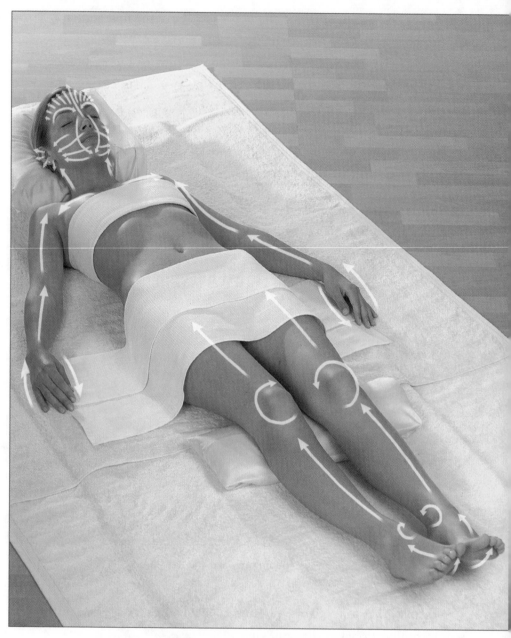

Sequence of an amber massage beginning at the feet
and ending at the forehead hairline

The Sequence of a
Harmonizing Massage with Amber

1. The chakra zones of the feet synchronously.
2. Back of the feet and ankles synchronously.
3. The right and left lower legs consecutively.
4. Knee joints synchronously.
5. The right and left thighs consecutively.
6. The right and left hands, inside and outside, consecutively.
7. Right and left forearms, up to the elbows, consecutively.
8. Each elbow joint, consecutively.
9. The right and left upper arm, up to the shoulder joint, consecutively.
10. Each shoulder joint, consecutively.
11. Shoulders and chest area.
12. The side and back of the neck.
13. The facial zones.
14. Let the client rest and enjoy the sensation.

This amber massage produces a feeling of circulating warmth in the body, with the result that too much or too little energy in the different body areas can be harmonized and balanced.

It's important to cleanse your stones following any type of massage. Amber loves a sunny place in twigs or tree cavities to "refuel." I also bathe it in a resonance bowl—simply pour water into the bowl, put the amber in it, and let the cleansing sounds resound.

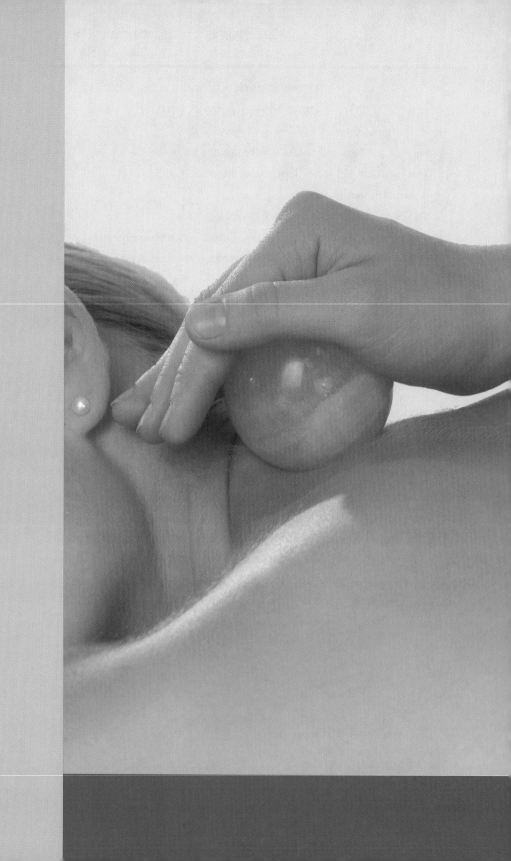

Part 5

Crystal Sphere Massage

■

By Ursula Dombrowsky

A massage with crystal spheres is a body-oriented treatment with wide-ranging effects. Massages coming from the spheres have an activating and relaxing effect at the same time, and they encourage a better body awareness, or coenesthesia.

THE INTERCONNECTEDNESS
OF THE BODY

The human body is a very complex organism. It consists of trillions of individual cells, and while we do not need to consciously regulate most functions—for example, blood circulation—we are still able to be aware of what is going on, even in our smallest toe. The body functions in a fascinating manner, and most of the time works very well, yet most of the time without being appreciated to any great degree.

A good metaphor is a business. In a small company with just a handful of employees, you can just imagine how much communication is necessary to make things work and be harmonious. You have to determine who is responsible for what, and regular meetings are necessary to ascertain the moment-by-moment status. Constant cooperation is necessary, and if just one person does not cooperate it has an effect on everyone. This becomes much more complicated if it's a very large company, with—in the body's case—trillions of "employees."

It is generally only when the body doesn't work efficiently that we come under pressure to do something. Maybe we have not taken notice of the subtle hints of small disorders, as we live our lives at such an active, hectic pace. There are so many ways to distract oneself . . . One thing is certain: we do not notice the small signs of disharmony early enough *if we are not in our own center.*

The Body's Three Systems of Communication

Communication between each of our trillions of cells happens in various ways and at different speeds. Blood circulation constitutes the slowest transportation. The entire hormonal system's messages, along with the white and red blood cells, clotting factors, and nutrients are all brought to the different areas of the body through the circulation of the blood. The oxygen that is transported in the blood is needed by each cell to be able to fulfill its function. It is jointly responsible for the burning of nutrients and for metabolic processes. Waste and carbon dioxide are also removed in the blood.

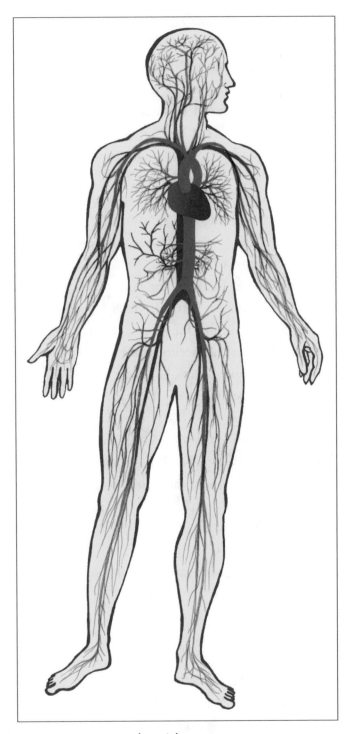

Arterial system

The nervous system also transmits information via electrical impulses that are transmitted to the individual cells extremely fast. You can perceive their speed when you burn your finger, for example. There are three types of nerve tissue: (1) the vegetative nerves that cause physical activity, such as gland or organ activity, at an unconscious level; (2) the motor nerves, which communicate motor impulses; and (3) the sensory nerves, which communicate sensation (touch, temperature, pain, etc.). Nerve fibers pervade the entire body in a similar way as the branches of a tree. They originate in the brain and run to the outer layers of our skin through the spinal cord.

The exit point of the fascicles (bundles of nerve fibers) is located between the respective vertebral bodies. An accumulation of ganglia is located next to the spine; from this the nerves then lead to the rest of the body and the extremities. Particular fascicles supply specific areas of the body. Each is responsible for an area of skin, a muscle area, and an organ system. If a blockage occurs in any one of those areas, it will show up in the other areas, too, in due course, because an altered nerve impulse now streams through the other supply areas.

The third information flow takes place in the meridian system. In Eastern medicine, such as Traditional Chinese medicine, these are energy channels that have been well known and used to heal since ancient times. The meridians are connected to certain organs, but they also pervade certain regions of the body. Information is always transmitted in both directions via the meridians. Scars and energetic blockages can disturb the energy flow there.

Finally, the body communicates through biophotons, which are light impulses (photons) of nonthermal origin in the visible and ultraviolet spectrum emitted from a biological system; they are responsible for direct cellular communication.

These three complex communications systems overlap in manifold ways and are deeply connected. This clearly demonstrates that no influence in the body remains only at the local level; it always spreads throughout the whole body, and finally reaches our soul, mind, and spirit.

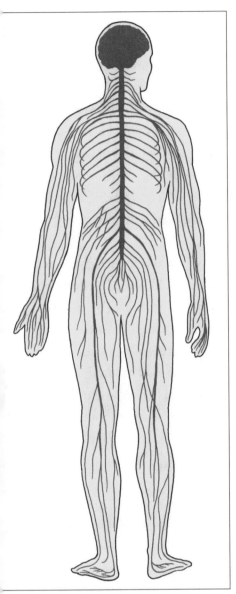

Nervous system

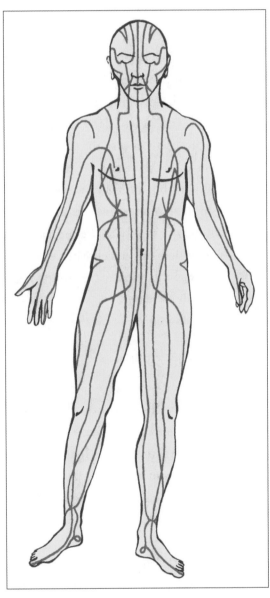

Meridian system

The Musculoskeletal System

An adult human has approximately 200 bones, and movement is possible due to the 277 twin and three single skeletal muscles that support them. The arbitrary skeletal muscles—the muscles that submit to our will and are attached to bone or joint via tendons—often reveal one's disposition. Muscle tone has a tendency to be too tight if a person is tense in general. Certainly the muscles will probably be tense somewhere if a person approaches something tensely; it usually shows up in the top part of the back (almost as if you've been carrying a heavy backpack), or similarly, if you've taken on a burden that's too heavy or you can't let go of daily affairs.

Physically, a certain hardheadedness shows up as a hard, tight neck. This often does not pertain to one's transient and changing body of thought, but rather to one's fundamental inner attitude. The muscles lose their suppleness if pain and tension are present. This means that the energy supply to the individual cells may decrease. Metabolic waste is then left in the cell, the cell's ability to exchange is reduced, and so on, until the result is that supplying the cell is made even more difficult.

This is where massage, particularly crystal massage, can be so helpful—but more on that later.

Spine and Pelvis

The spine is the axis of life. We walk upright and move thanks to its flexibility. It constitutes the middle point between the left and right sides of our body. The pelvis is the body's foundation, its horizontal center. An imbalance here has consequences for advancing (i.e., the legs), as well as for climbing or growing (i.e., the spine). This is why the pelvis and the spine play such an important role in massage with crystal spheres.

Body Rhythm

It is not just our inner attitudes that show up at the body level. Our environment and our activities also reflect what's happening in the

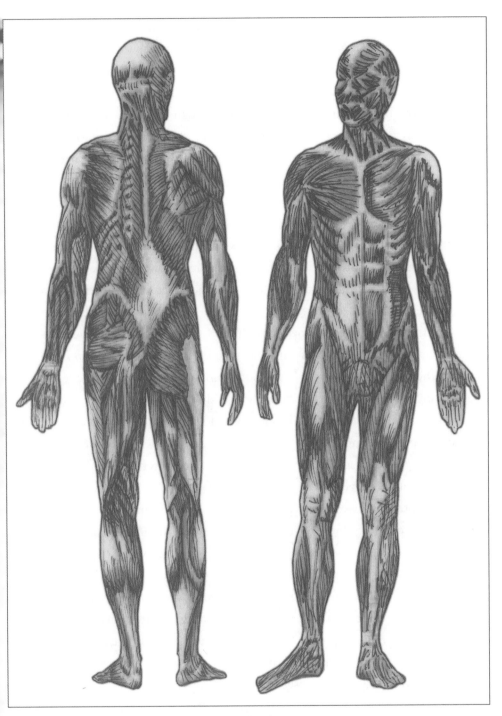

Musculoskeletal system

body. We do not, most of us, have the time anymore to live with a certain consistency, or in a more or less constant rhythm. Our sleeping behavior, for example, has been changed in a very definite way by the influence of the media and artificial lighting. As a result, oftentimes the body is unable to regenerate enough at night. Most people generally have a sleep rhythm that is too short; we also have not done enough spiritual preparatory work, because we have not taken time for reflection during the day. It is very good and helpful for sleep and therefore for the natural healing and regeneration processes of the body, if we find a way to review the day in the evening, before bedtime, without distraction, closing the things that have happened and becoming aware of what is still open. Then we do not have to take care of these reflections in our dreams, and the body receives more energy to regenerate itself because we are able to sleep better. This is the reason that the sleep that occurs before midnight is known as "beauty sleep"—it's because that period of time has to do with the detoxification and regeneration of the body. If the body cannot detoxify and regenerate optimally at night, it can result in residues and possible accumulation of toxic burdens. As a result, myogelosis (areas of hardening) can develop in the muscles. Again, these can be loosened effectively with regular massages and by drinking enough pure water—and, of course, with enough sleep.

Crystal massages are of great benefit when it comes to facilitating the interconnectedness of the body, as they can improve many different states of the body, mind, and spirit. The effects are long-lasting, however, only if they are incorporated into a healthy way of living, a gentle rhythm of life, a balanced diet, good sleep, flexible attitudes, and, last but not least, the pursuit of meaning and fulfilment in one's life. Massage with spheres especially can help things that need to be changed to flow again and can open up new perspectives so we can change and adapt consciously.

MY BACKGROUND IN CRYSTAL SPHERE MASSAGE

I have worked with various body-oriented techniques in my practice, including classical massage, spinal mobilization, meridian therapy, and energetic work. Crystal healing became part of my repertoire a few years ago when I was looking for a connection between these various disciplines. Crystal spheres came to my attention, and this massage developed out of my explorations with them. I received very good responses after just a few initial treatments. I found I could disperse tension very easily, and the body awareness, or coenesthesia, of my clients improved noticeably. Following treatment with the spheres, many clients became aware of amazing connections that allowed them to change lifelong habits. A reduction of previously held chronic tension was also a consequence of the work. I became very excited about the possibilities of incorporating these crystals into my practice.

In the beginning I worked with three different crystal spheres. Since then I have used fifty different types of crystal spheres. This variety has allowed me to make the massages more personal and directed.

CRYSTAL SPHERE TECHNIQUE

The most important motion when massaging using a crystal sphere is the horizontal figure eight. The figure eight is the symbol of infinity. In kinesiology it has a harmonizing effect on both halves of the brain by assisting the balancing of the left and right hemispheres. This figure eight consists of two complete circles that touch each other, each circle depicting a whole.

Figure eight

Take a sphere between your hands and rotate it to get a good feel for massaging with a crystal sphere. Notice how the sphere moves in your cupped hands. Then try it out for yourself by massaging your thigh, holding the sphere with a cupped hand. Vary the pressure and be aware of how this feels, and also what level of pressure you enjoy. We work with adjusted pressure in physical massage; this means that we go up to a bearable threshold of pressure before we hit actual pain. More pressure is usually possible than one can imagine.

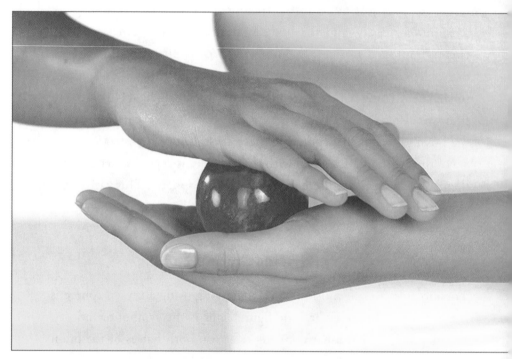

Rotate a sphere between your hands
to become familiar with this crystal shape.

THE CRYSTAL SPHERE MASSAGE SEQUENCE

In this treatment, the client is massaged by applying varied pressure in different directions using a crystal sphere. The massage is administered over the whole of the back, beginning at the hip areas, adapting the pressure as dictated by the situation and the person. The whole body can be massaged in this manner as well with a little practice. Muscles are relaxed and circulation is encouraged through massage with crystal spheres, which have an activating and relaxing effect at the same time, and encourage a better body awareness, or coenesthesia, resulting in distinctly increased vitality. Physical blockages, along with their mental and spiritual origins can also be released in this fashion.

A physical blockage can have many causes. Sometimes it simply develops out of excessive demand on physical capabilities; often, however, emotional and spiritual issues underlie the problem. In the long run, it is not sufficient to treat the person only on one level. This is where massage that incorporates crystal spheres can be so effective, as good therapy always addresses the person in her entirety, identifying and working with the flow of energy between spirit/soul, mind, and body. Nevertheless, the emphasis is clearly on the physical body in massaging with crystal spheres, as blockages that have been held by the body for a long time are easily found using this method. This has far-reaching holistic effects. When attention is directed to the body, with the help of the crystals, the body's distinct language can tell us what the human "computer" has been programmed with by the mind. By becoming aware of these kinds of connections between body, mind, and spirit/soul and addressing them through crystal massage, we can really make big changes and improvements on all levels.

A warm, quiet room that smells good is best for the massage. You can give it on the floor or on a massage table; the more comfortable the position, the more enjoyable the massage. The person being massaged should only be wearing underpants. Cover the person for comfort as needed. Having the room warm enough facilitates relaxation. Massage with spheres is performed directly on the skin, so massage oil is not needed, because the massage is more effective without oil.

To begin, the person lies on her front to have her back massaged. It sometimes feels more comfortable if a pillow is placed under the stomach, which results in relaxation of the lumbar region and the small of

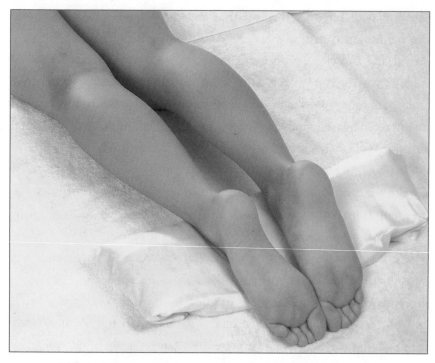

When the person is lying on her front, a rolled-up towel
placed under the ankles may increase comfort.

the back. This position is important if a heavy lordosis (curvature of
the spine to the front) exists. A rolled-up towel or a blanket can be
placed under the ankles, if necessary.

Any crystal that is available as a sphere is suitable to use when massaging. A sphere with a diameter of between three and five centimeters
(approximately one to two inches) is adequate. The smaller the sphere,
the smaller the area being massaged and the less pressure needed.
When using a larger sphere the skin area and the receptors under it are
touched more superficially. If you would like to try this out on yourself,
then press down on your skin with the tip of your finger, and then, in
comparison, with the entire surface of your thumb. Feel the difference?

The most effective massage always comes as a result of being totally
present for the person you are working on, with the intention that you
are acting as a catalyst for improving her health. That said, there is

Selecting a Sphere

There are various ways of selecting the appropriate crystal sphere. You can approach it in a playful manner if you have more than one to choose from. And if you only have one sphere, just use this one. But if you have more than one sphere to choose from, it might be good if the person you are massaging selects her crystal, because it is her body that is going to be treated. The person might find which crystal is right by holding a hand over the spheres with eyes closed. This feeling might show up in the form of a tickling sensation, a feeling of warmth, of coolness, or simply by the person touching the right crystal. The desire to select a certain sphere will simply be there. Another possibility is that the person selects the sphere that appeals to her most at that moment. You can also attach a number to each of your spheres (or line them up, left to right) and ask the person to give you a number, then simply take the corresponding sphere. Or you could offer to choose the sphere for the person you are going to massage yourself. To do this you can refer to the crystal information that follows at the end of this part of the book.

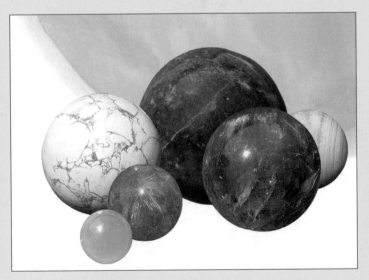

Any crystal available as a sphere can be used to perform a massage.

no sense in taking over the blockages or problems of another person. Everyone is responsible for his or her own life, and also for making life changes. The body can often regulate a physical disorder after an external impulse has set events in motion. That is why it is good if you remain aware of yourself and your boundaries and aim simply to be quietly present.

Establish a protective boundary around yourself and the person you are massaging. There are various ways you can do this:

- Through words, by saying a prayer or a protective phrase
- By visualizing yourself wrapped in light (white, violet, etc.)
- By using aromatic or Aura-Soma oils, for example—putting them on your hands and then moving your hands over and around your body and your client's without actually touching it in order to create a protective shield
- By tapping your hands before the massage and becoming more aware of your own body in this way

Having done your own personal preparation and protection, you can then tune in to the person lying in front of you.

Start by standing or sitting next to the left-hand side of the person to be treated and establishing contact.

The massage begins in the pelvic area. You experiment with pressure levels here; be sure to give enough time and attention to this area. The more you can bring balance to this area, the easier it will be to continue and develop the massage. Work with an appropriate degree of pressure in the introductory part of the massage. It is sometimes necessary to apply pressure right up to the pain threshold when freeing blockages, but never go over it. A steady increase in pressure is more enjoyable than starting off the massage with heavy pressure; remember to always apply a suitable amount of pressure during this stage of the crystal sphere massage.

The whole hand guides the sphere, with palm and fingers used

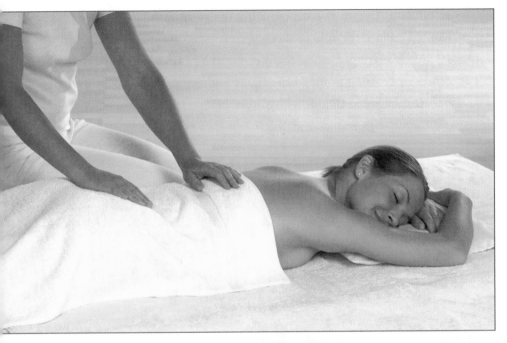

Establishing contact

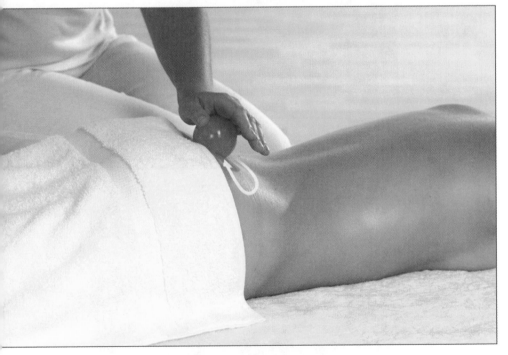

Introduction at the pelvic area

in tandem. Guide the sphere with the right hand (if you are right-handed). Place the sphere carefully onto the sacrum. The hip and dorsal area is massaged using the motion of a horizontal figure eight. The center or crossing point of the figure eight is always located in the spinal area, between the individual vertebrae.

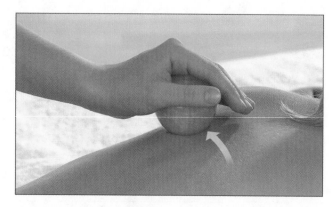

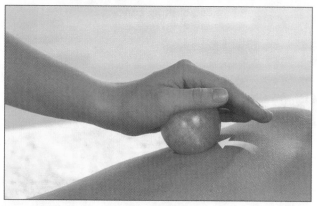

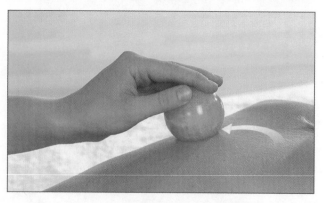

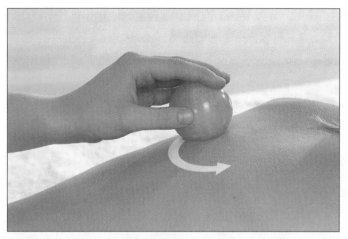

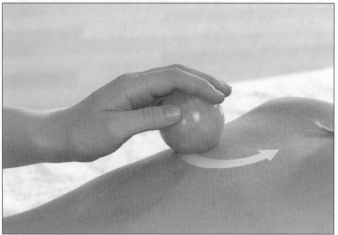

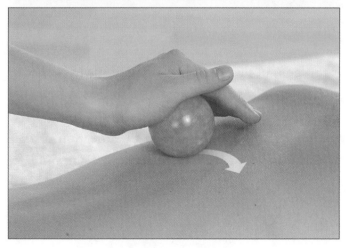

Guiding the sphere with your hand

The buttock muscles are then massaged firmly, between five and seven times. The sphere can also be guided in circles in this area. A good level of pressure is appropriate here because the buttock muscles usually contain a buildup of tension.

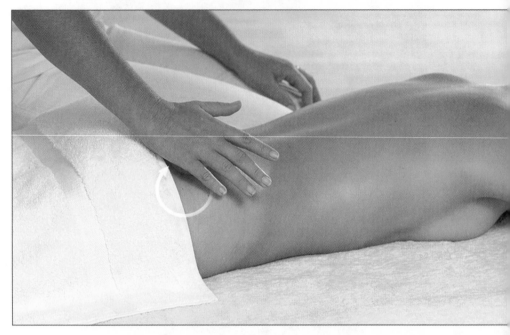

Firm massage of the buttock muscles

Then return to the bottom of the back and massage in figure-eight movements again. Work up the entire spine in figure eights, making sure that the loops of the eight always cross at the individual vertebrae. It is important to adapt the pressure here so that it feels good to the person being massaged.

The entire spine is worked over in the direction of the cervical vertebrae this way. The goal is to balance the right and left sides of the body.

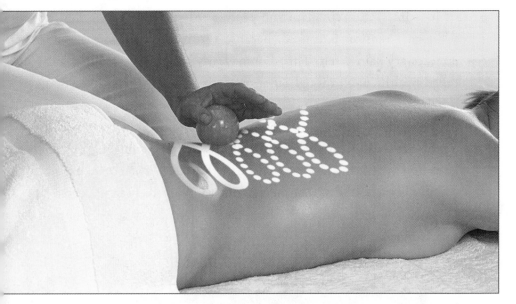

Working up the spine with figure-eight motion

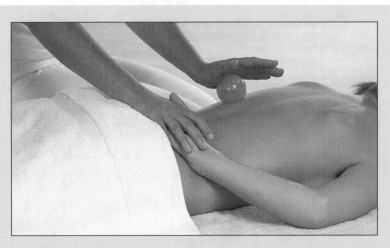

Tickle stop

A little trick that can help if someone turns out to be ticklish is to take her hand and place it on her back. The person then feels as if the treatment is being carried out by her own hand—and tickling yourself just doesn't work.

It is important to adapt the pressure of the massage so that no additional tension is caused, because the person will stiffen up if unnecessary pain is felt. This should clearly be avoided. There is a so-called healthy pain, though, that, while it hurts, also helps the body to relax.

Next, massage next to the spinal column and over the back muscles on the left side, starting from the neck area. Use a circling motion that leads downward, in the direction of the hip area. The circles are not large, only three to five centimeters (one to two inches) in diameter.

Once you have arrived at the hip, massage up the spinal column, again in figure eights.

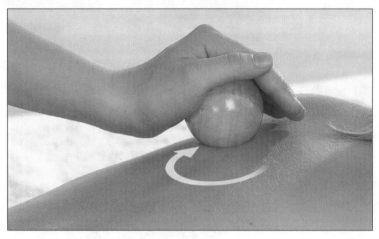

Massaging the back muscles on the left side

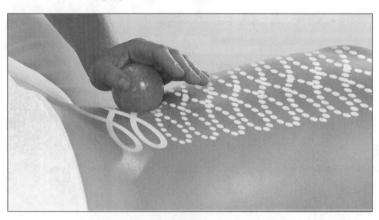

The figure-eight motions

Massage the muscles on the right side of the back using the same circular motions you used on the left side of the body.

Now massage the side muscles. You can apply firm pressure near the shoulder blades, but a lighter touch is required between the ribs.

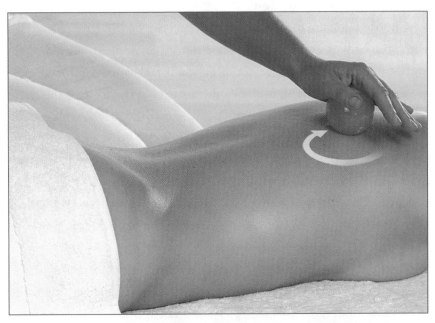

Massaging the muscles on the right side of the back

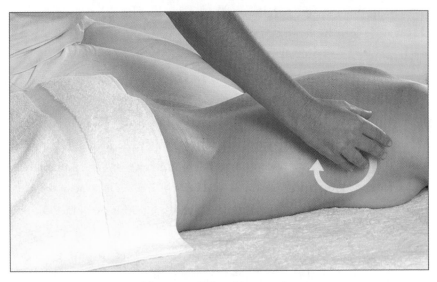

Massage of the side muscles

It is easier to massage the shoulder area if you change your position. Stand or sit at the top of the body; this enables you to work on this area systematically. Take your time here and massage the entire shoulder area, using small circles. Adapt the pressure here as well, so that it is perceived as having a loosening effect.

Choose a posture for yourself that means you do not have to massage with your arm at an angle. The pressure is then applied more directly and can be administered better, plus you'll feel more comfortable.

Continue from the shoulder to the muscles at the nape of the neck, which are also massaged at length, to little by little loosen what can be strong tension in this area.

Until now the spheres have been guided in your cupped hand. There is a different grip for the next, more energetic part of the massage. The sphere is now placed on the spinal column and is held between the thumb and index finger, using the bent middle finger to guide it.

Position yourself on the right side of your client. Starting at the nape of the neck, the middle finger now pushes the sphere down the back slowly and lightly. When you reach the hip level, lift the sphere and replace at the nape of the neck next to the spine, and roll it down to the hip once again, parallel to the first roll. The sphere is rolled in this way, length by length, until the entire width of the back has been treated.

Note that this energetic work on the back is always carried out in the direction of the meridians, in the direction of the legs.

The sphere helps to activate energy flow in the direction it is moved in, and you will be able to see where energy is still blocked. The movement of the rolling sphere can change strongly here: it can move lightly and freely, become inhibited and slow down, or even appear to stop. Experiencing these sensations requires a certain amount of practice, but they can be very exact indicators of where energy is blocked. It is good to repeat the massage of blocked areas or areas where the energy is not flowing freely several times. The energetic rolling from the neck in the

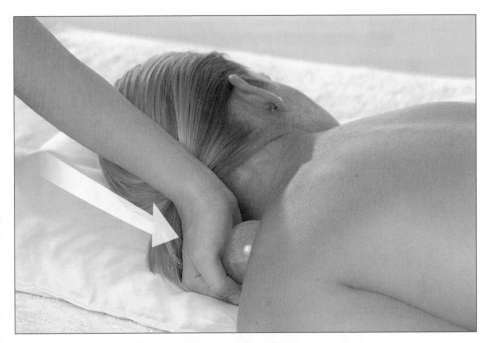

Massage of the shoulder

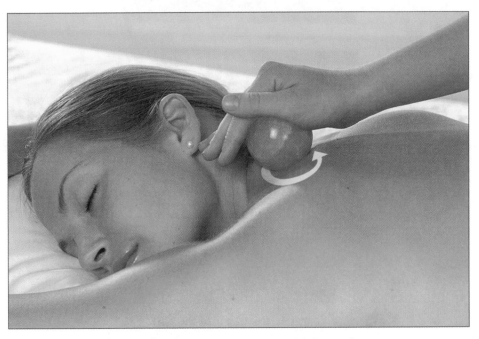

Dissolving tension at the nape of the neck

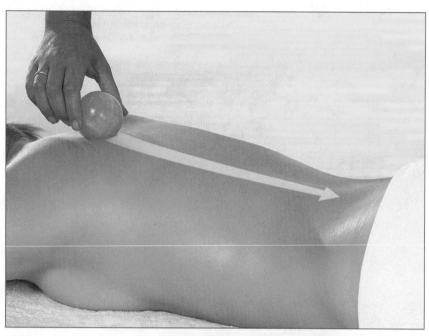

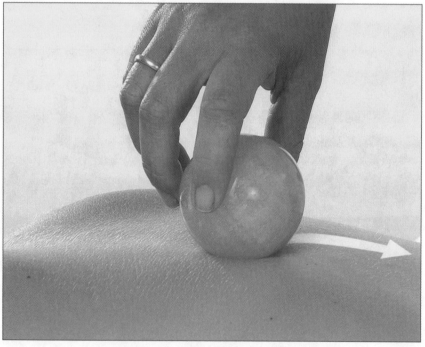

Energetic treatment of the back

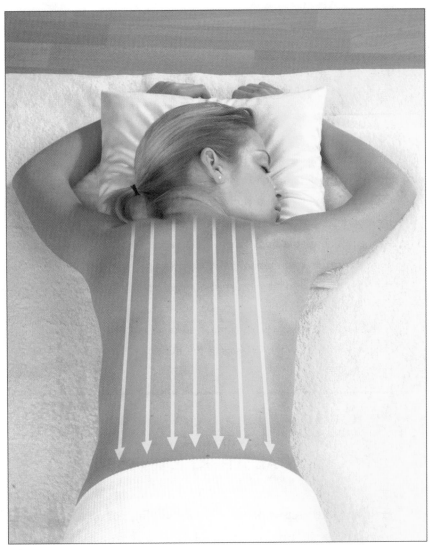

Massage down the back toward the legs

direction of the buttocks should be repeated and the results monitored. You can end the treatment as soon as the sphere rolls smoothly at the point where it was sticking, or you can continue, letting your intuition guide you in massage of other areas of the body. A creative game develops between sphere and user—always for the well-being of the person being treated.

A Few
Points to Remember

+ The massage should be administered in a quiet, constant, gentle rhythm, one that enables your client to relax on the one hand, yet stimulates circulation on the other.

+ It is possible to massage the whole body, but be very careful in the abdominal area. It is important that you take into account the position of the colon, which begins in the lower right abdomen, then ascends on the right and runs across to the left side of the abdomen between the navel and the solar plexus. It descends down the left-hand side of the body. This is the reason we always massage in a clockwise direction when we work on the abdomen; this assists the flow of movement through the intestines. The abdominal area is the area where deep feelings are situated; this means that a lot of feelings can arise when we massage the abdomen. This is why I recommend that when massaging the abdominal area only a very light pressure is used.

BENEFITS OF
CRYSTAL SPHERE MASSAGE

Massage with crystal spheres is very good for relaxing muscles and for encouraging blood circulation in the tissues. This can appear as a feeling of warmth, a tingling, or even a feeling of lightness. A pleasant feeling of heaviness can also develop—you get a sense of the body and what it needs. Rotating the sphere allows you to massage with stronger pressure, so that deeper muscle layers can also enjoy the massage. Therefore massage with crystal spheres is both liberating and loosening. This type of massage is very helpful in cases of tension (of an acute or chronic nature), inner feelings of stress, fatigue, muscle cramps, backaches, after a hectic day, as something good to do for a partner, as a health precaution, and for many similar reasons or related conditions.

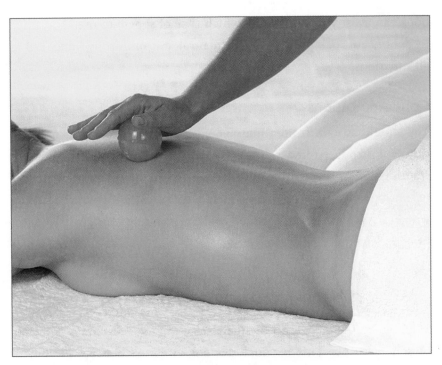

Crystal sphere massage is a very effective technique
for relaxation and energy balance.

Massaging with spheres also encourages the balancing of the left and right sides of the body. Different aspects are attributed to these two sides. The right side represents the masculine principle: intellectual, active, future-oriented. It also suggests authoritativeness, assertiveness, and goal-orientation. The left side represents the feminine, nurturing nature: intuition, the past, patience, and an ability to relate to people and situations. We can work with both our intuition and our intellect if the right and left side of the body are in harmony. A blockage can also build up just on one side of the body, either the emotional or the intellectual side, depending on our inner attitude. We always treat both sides of the body when giving a crystal massage.

Finally, and significantly, the benefits of a crystal sphere massage will be determined by the type of sphere/stone that is selected. The compendium of crystal spheres located at the end of this part of the book can assist you in deciding which type of sphere to use. And when in doubt, use rock crystal, as it is neutral and uniformly beneficial in all situations.

Contraindications

You should abstain from a massage with spheres if strong, acute pain exists; if strong pain develops suddenly, after a jerky movement; if transmission or perception disorders exist in the extremities; in the case of open wounds; or immediately after surgery. If you are not sure whether it is appropriate to give a massage, consult your client's doctor or complementary practitioner.

A COMPENDIUM OF CRYSTAL SPHERES

I am including here only a small selection of the stones available in sphere shape. This list includes any effects and reactions I have observed. This is definitely not a comprehensive list but should help to differentiate the focal point of the spheres and assist the reader in beginning to assemble a crystal sphere massage collection.

A distinct connection between the type and locality of existing tension and other problems, and an intuitively chosen crystal has long been established. You can basically use any crystal that is available as a sphere. People always find the stone suitable for them. But this guide should serve well in guiding the reader toward a specific desired result.

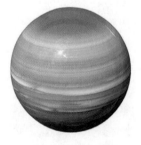

Agate imparts the wonderful awareness of one's skin being a protective covering. It is soft and comforting. Agate assists in building up protection and helps you to help yourself. It brings a feeling of security, allowing you to let go. Agate fortifies, strengthens, and helps you work better under pressure.

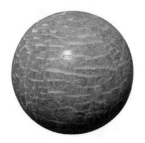

Amazonite is very helpful if you have too many burdens, resulting in tension and pain. It helps the body find peace. It has a relaxing and pain-relieving effect.

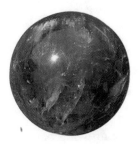

Amethyst is very effective for tension. It loosens cramped muscles and can also be used to treat headaches. It has a relaxing and rather cooling effect, which is why it can be very helpful after overexertion.

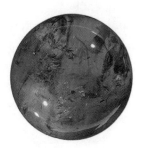

Ametrine imparts a beautiful sense of harmony to the body. It calms nerves and brings inner peace, while simultaneously making you feel awake and lively. It brings exactly the right balance between tension and relaxation. Ametrine has a strongly uplifting effect and can therefore be useful at times of unhappiness, tension, or discontentment.

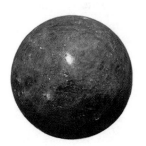

Apatite can be very useful for physical exhaustion. It has a strengthening and constructive effect. It can be helpful for posture disorders and is good for bones and joints.

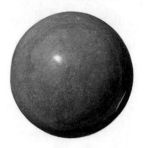

Aventurine is good if the skin is sensitive or irritated. It can also help mentally if you are irritated, nervous, anxious, and tormented by constantly circling thoughts. It can also be used when lack of rest from stress has resulted in blockages in the body.

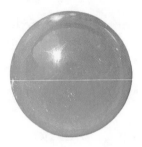

Calcite (orange) is a sunny, strengthening crystal that gives very good coenesthesia and strengthens one's acceptance of oneself. It tightens tissue, mobilizes muscles, and strengthens bones. Calcite is also good for massaging children who have growing pains.

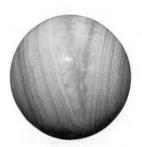

Chalcedony as a blue-banded crystal offers assistance to the body in getting everything flowing again. It is also appropriate for tightness of the skin. It lightens the spirits and stimulates conversation.

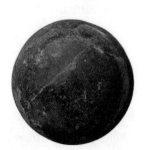

Chrysocolla has a balancing effect and is harmonizing for all areas of the body. It brings intellect and intuition into harmony, balances mood fluctuation, and smooths muscles, tissues, and skin. It is also very good for the healing of scar tissue. Chrysocolla can also be stimulating for the digestive system if the hip and buttock areas are massaged well.

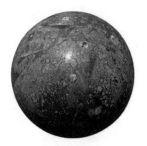

Epidote is a very good crystal for fatigue, especially fatigue caused by long illness or mental strain. Therefore a very good constructive and strengthening massage can be given with it.

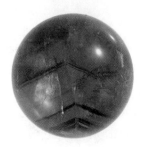

Fluorite makes you physically and mentally agile: it loosens energetic blockages, clears the head, and is good for joints, bones, cartilage, tissue, and skin. This is why fluorite can support you if you are trying to change your posture.

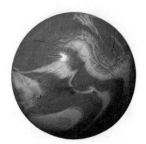

Jasper, especially in its red crystal form, has an inspiring, strengthening, and vitalizing effect. It helps to support and strengthen you if you are going through a difficult time. Jasper stimulates blood circulation and warms you if you have a tendency to feel cold. A massage with this crystal is activating, so it is better not to use it for a massage too late in the evening.

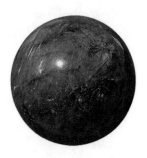

Labradorite has a cooling effect if you are hot-tempered and a warming effect if you are too cool. It frees the tissues of waste and sediment and therefore also helps rheumatic pain. Labradorite helps you to become aware of the origins of any physical disorders.

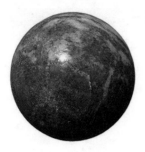

Lapis lazuli makes you open, self-assured, and self-confident. It gives you a sense of space if you feel constricted, allowing the body to be calm but responsive. Lapis lazuli can stimulate you to hold inspiring conversations after a massage with it!

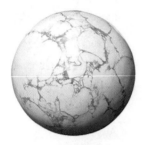

Magnesite relaxes, calms, and eases cramps. It is good for the muscles and connective tissue in a crystal sphere massage. Magnesite helps you to let go and eases headaches. It can also be used as part of a detoxification regime.

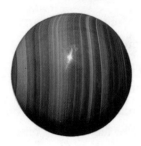

Malachite is particularly good for women, as it relieves cramps and works on menstrual problems. It makes sense to massage intensively with this sphere in the lumbar and sacral bone area for these problems. Malachite brings back memories and therefore helps one realize the cause of existing blockages.

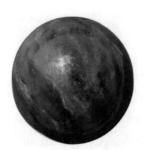

Nephrite is a good crystal to strengthen the kidneys; this will show up in a better flow of energy. It helps the body to thoroughly detoxify.

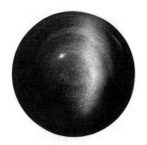

Obsidian is very good for pain; it also helps after trauma or an operation, either to heal after surgery or after consultation with a doctor! Massage with obsidian loosens energetic blockages.

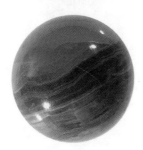

Ocean agate (ocean jasper) is very good for a constructive massage. It has an uplifting and motivating effect and is very good for engendering strength and peace in hectic times, or after an illness.

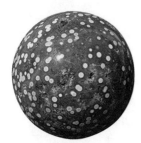

Onyx marble (aragonite) is very good for strain and makes one loose-limbed and aware of one's body. Onyx marble helps in disorders of the back, spine, and vertebrae. It is important to position the patient correctly when massaging with onyx marble (put a pillow under the stomach). Pressure has to be applied very carefully in the spinal area.

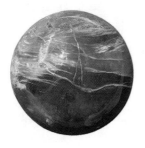

Petrified wood helps you feel a general sense of well-being, both within your body and in the external world. Petrified wood improves your relationship with your body; it can sometimes help if someone is overweight and at times when you do not like yourself. It has a warming effect, and is therefore good for cold limbs.

Rhodonite is a very good crystal with which to massage scar tissue. It can help the tissue become smoother again. It also helps one be more motivated and active.

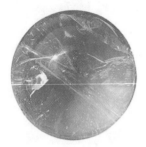

Rock crystal can be used very effectively in any situation. It has a vitalizing and harmonizing effect on both the left and right halves of the body. Because of its strengthening effect it can help you become more conscious of your body.

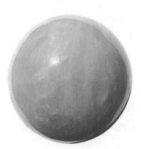

Rose quartz is a good crystal for harmonious and affectionate treatments. It allows the body to be calm and relaxed and encourages one's awareness.

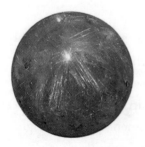

Rutilated quartz has a liberating and vitalizing effect, especially for the chest and heart area if you massage the upper back intensively. It can therefore be used when one feels constricted. Rutilated quartz stimulates the regeneration of tissues and therefore helps in chronic health conditions.

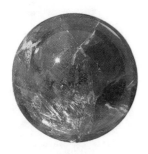

Smoky quartz is a good aid if there is tension in the back area that needs to be dispersed. It is very effective as an anti-stress crystal.

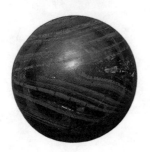

Stromatolite has a very good effect on the digestion. Massage the bottom part of the back intensively to help the digestion in this way; as it helps one to let go, it has a detoxifying effect.

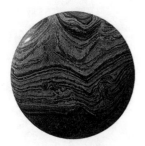

Tiger iron gives vitality and energy for life. It encourages blood circulation and haematopoiesis and helps with extreme fatigue. Tiger iron lets you feel vigorous and strong again. It is better not to massage with tiger iron too late in the evening, though; its effects are so stimulating that you might not be able to sleep.

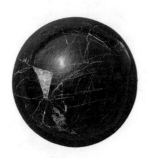

Tourmaline (black schorl) is very good for the energy flow through the nerves, which is why it can be used to improve body sensations. It can also be used to treat scar tissue; however, it can take repeated massages to accomplish this.

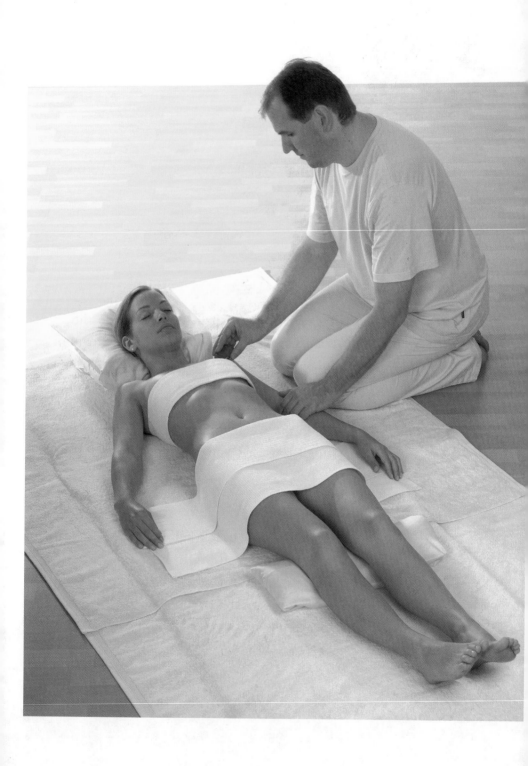

About the Authors

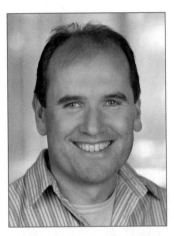

MICHAEL GIENGER

Michael Gienger (1964–2014) was known as an author, editor, and publisher of works dealing with natural studies, philosophy, and healing, especially crystal healing. He worked as a shiatsu masseur before he became involved in crystal healing at the end of the 1980s. Massaging with crystals was part of his life for thirty years, and he shared his experiences and knowledge in seminars and training courses for twenty years. This work is now being continued by his colleagues in the Cairn Elen Life Schools.

Michael Gienger was joint founder of the Stuttgart Crystal Healing Research Group (1988), Steinheilkunde e.V. (1995), the Cairn Elen Life Schools (1997), and the Cairn Elen Crystal Healing Network (1998). From 1997 to 2002 he was involved with the project Minerals in Medical Science, which brought together science and the healing experience. Michael Gienger was well known for several books he published in English: *Crystal Power, Crystal Healing* (Cassell Illustrated, 1998); *Healing Crystals* (Earthdancer/Findhorn Press, 2005), *Crystal Massage for Health and Healing* and *The Healing Crystal First Aid Manual* (Earthdancer/Findhorn Press, both 2006); and *Healing Stones for the Vital Organs* (with Wolfgang Maier; Healing Arts Press, 2009).

You can learn more about Michael Gienger and his projects at the following German websites:

www.michael-gienger.de
www.cairn-elen.de
www.edelstein-massagen.de
www.steinheilkunde-ev.de

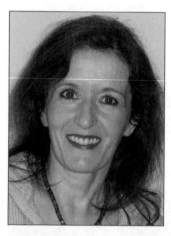

HILDEGARD WEISS

Hildegard Weiss lives and works at the Crystal Healing Centre in Grünebach, Germany. She enjoys encouraging people to live in accordance with nature and offers lectures, workshops, and courses, as well as health counseling with Bach flowers and astrology. Relaxing massages that further awareness of our body and its needs and that are attuned to the individual client are standard parts of her repertoire. Her knowledge comes from many years of study with Michael Gienger (crystal healing), Dr. Wighart Strehlow (the teachings of Hildegard von Bingen), and Daniel Agustoni (craniosacral therapy), as well as other teachers of crystal healing, massage, and natural healing. Her desire is to show people that a mindful interaction with their body, mind, and spirit results in more joie de vivre, more bliss.

Hildegard Weiss has been instructed and supported on her path of practice by her Buddhist sangha in Hohenau, Bavaria, who live by the guidelines of the Zen master Thich Nhat Hanh. Training in this practice is also offered at the Crystal Healing Centre.

More information about programs, seminars, and lectures is available by writing her at:

PRISMA, Hildegard Weiss
Hauptstrasse 7

57520 Grünebach, Germany
phone: +49 2741 22218
fax: +49 2741 932 9485
prismaww@hotmail.com
www.prismazentrum.de

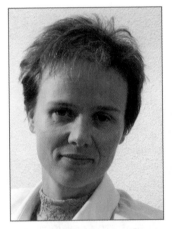

URSULA DOMBROWSKY

Ursula Dombrowsky has a diploma in medical massage and reflexology. She has been fascinated by crystals since childhood and has immersed herself in this field since her first crystal healing seminar in 1998. Today her practice combines crystal healing with manual and energetic physical and speech therapy.

Ursula Dombrowsky started crystal healing courses for children during her three years of study at the Cairn Elen Life School. Her first book, *Wenn Steine erzählen* [When Crystals Tell Stories] (Neue Erde Verlag, 2003) grew out of this, along with her experience with her crystal-enthusiast daughters.

Apart from her work as masseuse and therapist with her own practice, Ursula Dombrowsky offers crystal healing seminars and training in which she teaches massage with crystal spheres, morphic field massage, and other crystal healing topics. Her crystal healing elementary and main trainings conform to the guidelines of Michael Gienger and the Cairn Elen Life Schools.

You can contact her at:

Ursula Dombrowsky, Büelgass 26,
8625 Gossau, Switzerland
phone and fax: +41 1936 2114
ursula@dombrowsky.ch
www.dombrowsky.ch

Index

Page numbers in *italics* represent illustrations.